Basi

Calculations

For Nurses, Emergency and Perioperative Practitioners.

John England

Table of Contents

Disclaimer

The author has made every effort to ensure that the contents of this book are correct, error free, and a reasonable representation of the design goal, which is to present techniques and examples for calculating drug dosages. This body of work should be regarded as a text book for learning purposes, and not a clinical manual.

No responsibility or liability for damages caused by any erroneous contents of this book are accepted and, in all situations, recommends that professional guidelines, national policies, and direction from suitably qualified medical staff, take precedence over the information contained herein.

Preface

Drug administration is a principle factor in the delivery of most non-minor patient care, and the ability to persistently and reliably calculate drug dosages is essential, if drug efficacy and, more significantly, patient safety is to be ensured.

Registered and licensed healthcare practitioners, such as nurses, paramedics, and anaesthetic technicians, have both a professional obligation and moral duty to ensure that a particular drug dosage has been correctly metered, and performing those necessary drug calculations is something which patients expect as a matter of routine, and performed with a high degree of accuracy.

Drug calculations vary in their levels of complexity, and this book focuses on some of the simpler and more commonly encountered types of problem, using short equations or step-by-step sequences for each calculation type. In all cases, the key skill for calculating drug doses is transposition of fractions and simple equations, as taught at Primary school level. Once transposition is understood, finding the unknown value in a dosage problem becomes just a matter of routine - there is no mystery to it.

<u>Note</u>: More worked examples can be found in the accompanying book – *Drug Calculation Workbook* (Amazon Publishing).

For more advanced calculation types, such as moles, infusions, and alligations, refer to *Advanced Drug Calculations* (Amazon Publishing).

Introduction

Basic Drug Calculations is composed of short chapters, each of which addresses a specific and typical type of calculation problem.

These calculations include some of the most commonly encountered types of problem, which anyone working in healthcare should become proficient at solving.

The calculation types include:

- ► Unit conversions

- ► Body Mass Index

- ► Body Surface Area

- ► Tablet and Ampoule dosages

- ► Giving set drip rates

- ► Pumped infusions

- ► Displacement volumes

- ► Drug w/v concentrations
- ► Dilutions

To consolidate the calculation explanations, a comprehensive test is given, and worked answers are provided. The test is not meant to be a pass or fail exercise; instead, it should be considered a demonstration model for the types of problem which should be mastered, and a prompt for continuing practice.

By mastering this presentation of commonly found drug calculation examples, the reader can expect to gain confidence in one of the most important foundations of healthcare delivery – pharmacology calculations.

Tip: By repeatedly re-reading this book with, say, two months between each revisit, recognition of the different types of drug calculation problem will become more obvious, and recalling the relevant formula (equation) types will become automatic which, together, will instill confidence because, as they say, practice makes perfect.

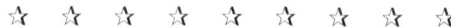

Measurement Systems

The uncoordinated history of measurement systems matches the historical isolation between different parts of the world, where different methods were developed to provide reference values, particularly for weight (more correctly, mass) and distance.

As trade expanded between different societies, and the sharing of scientific findings became more widespread, the idea for a standardised system of measurements developed, with impetus and suggestions from disparate sources.

The first record of a suggestion for such a standardised system is that of Bishop John Wilkins, in 1668, who promoted the concept of decimalisation, which means using measuring systems with units of ten, rather than, for example, dividing one foot into twelve inches, or fourteen pounds to make a stone, and so forth. His idea - a "universal measure" system – was published, but not acted upon – it was seen more as a theoretical proposition, rather than the real proposal which he intended.

In 1670, a French priest, Gabriel Mouton, also promoted the decimal idea, but nothing came of this, until 1795, when Prieur de la Cote d'Or, also in France, introduced the idea of describing sub-division prefixes for measurement systems, using "deci" and "centi", among others. At about the same time, an early form of the metric system was starting to gain acceptance in several parts of France, but this was quashed by Napoleon Bonaparte, who preferred a modified system, which he thought best suited French commerce.

In the United States, during the late eighteenth century, Thomas Jefferson proposed the replacement of the set of Imperial measurements with ones based on the metric system, but others deemed that such a radical change was unnecessary, because American commerce, and society, were doing well with the Imperial system, so it was retained although, since the 1990's, the adoption of the S.I. system has started to replace the Imperial system in the areas of science and engineering.

After Napoleon, the idea of a universal measuring system regained popularity in France, and the French became the champions of its benefits, adopting the metric system of measurement in the mid 19th century.

Now, the metric system is part of the *Système International d'Unités*, or S.I. - used in all areas of science, including pharmacology.

The Metric System

For calculation purposes, the advantage of the metric system is, to some degree, counter-balanced by the ease of which mistakes can occur, due to the misplacement of decimal points, by confusing, for example, "milli" and "micro". Additionally, the rules for expressing values are rarely followed, or understood, and that leads to errors.

Some of the terminology rules include:

√ Use singular abbreviations; "ml", not "mls".

√ Always place a blank space between the unit and value; "10 mg", not "10mg".

√ Do not abbreviate unit prefixes which denote very small, or very large values; use "microgram", not "mcg".

√ Unit prefixes which are not abbreviated, such as "nanogram", should be written in the singular, when denoting particular values (25 nanogram), but written in the plural, when used in a general context, such as in "The supply needed is in nanograms".

Unit abbreviations:

Unit	Abbreviation?
Litre	L or l
Millilitre	ml
Microlitre	microlitre
Mole	mol
Millimole	mmol
Micromole	micromol
Gram	g
Milligram	mg
Microgram	microgram
Nanogram	nanogram

Another clinically acceptable abbreviation is *gtt* (guttae), which signifies a giving set's drops per ml. If "gtt" were not used, it would be more likely that *drops/ml* could be confused with *drops/min*, which could produce the obvious result of a calculation error so, using "gtt", in the context of drug calculations, reducing the chance of misinterpretation and is, therefore, an aid to safety. Naturally, if "gtt" is used outside of the context of using a giving set, it is much more likely to be the abbreviation for *glucose tolerance test*, so always ensure its use is in the right context.

Prefixes

With respect to drug administration, the extremes of values, large and small, are rarely needed but, for completeness, some of the more extreme value prefixes are given here:

Prefix	Value
Giga	1,000,000,000
Mega	1,000,000
Kilo	1,000
Hecto	100
Deka	10
Deci	1 divided by 10
Centi	1 divided by 100
Milli	1 divided by 1,000
Micro	1 divided by 1,000,000
Nano	1 divided by 1,000,000,000
Pico	1 divided by 1,000,000,000,000

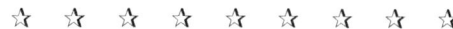

Système International d'Unités

The SI model, which was agreed and adopted at the General Conference on Weights and Measures, in Paris, in 1960, is composed of definitions of seven different measurement categories (see table below).

The SI system includes some aspects of the metric system, specifically the kilogram and metre, but the metric and SI systems should not be confused. The metric system defines units which have an immediate and practical purpose for measurement. The SI system, on the other hand, defines what measure systems, for particular applications, are to be considered as "standard".

Confusion over metric and SI systems is commonly seen in publications where, for example, the claim is made that the litre is the SI unit of volume, the gram is the SI unit of mass, and the pascal is the SI unit for pressure when, in fact, the pascal and litre are SI *derived* units, and the SI unit of mass is the kilogram - not the gram.

The seven SI units:

Dimension	*Unit*
Length	*Metre*
Mass	*Kilogram*
Time	*Second*
Electrical current	*Ampere*
Temperature	*Kelvin*
Amount of a substance	*Mole*
Light intensity	*Candela*

Unit Conversions

When dealing with calculations, values should always be converted to the same measurement system and domain, such as converting imperial pounds to kilograms, and ensuring variables measured in micrograms are not included in the same calculation as variables measured in milligrams, for example.

Another recommended practice is to avoid expressing variables in decimals and, instead, convert the value to a smaller type; for example, instead of using 0.0475 mg, multiply by 1,000 to form 47.5 microgram.

To be fully proficient at unit conversions, specifically in the metric system, some basic rules of unit division and discrimination must be mastered. Specifically, with respect to prefixes for canonical units, such as the gram or litre.

Commonly used prefixes

Prefix	Meaning
Mega	Unit * million
Kilo	Unit * thousand
Deci	One tenth unit
Centi	One hundredth
Milli	One thousandth
Micro	One millionth
Nano	One billionth
Pico	One trillionth

◄ *Example 1*

Convert 5' 3" to its metric equivalent.

◄◄◄ Solution ►►►

- ◆ Convert 5' to inches: 5 * 12 = 60 inch.

- ◆ Add 3 = 63 inch.

- ◆ 1 inch = 2.5 cm, so 63 * 2.5 = 157.5 cm.

Answer: 157.5 cm.

✎ *Example 2*

How many microlitres are there in one centilitre?

◄◄◄ Solution ►►►

- ◆ One centilitre is 1 litre/100 = 10 ml.

- ◆ 1 ml = 1,000 microlitre.

- ◆ 10 ml * 1,000 = 10,000 microlitre.

Answer: 10,000 microlitre.

✎ *Example 3*

What is the total mass of drug T, in mg, of 40 tablets, each of which contains 150 microgram?

◄◄◄ Solution ►►►

- ◆ 40 * 150 = 6,000 microgram.

- ◆ 6,000 microgram/1,000 = 6 mg.

Answer: 6 mg.

✑ *Example 4*

Convert 0.075 g to micrograms.

◄◄◄ Solution ►►►

- ◆ Convert 0.075 g to mg: 0.075 * 1,000 = 75 mg.

- ◆ Convert 75 mg to microgram: 75 * 1,000 75,000.

Answer: 0.075 g = 75,000 microgram.

Body Mass Index

BMI is a descriptive measurement of a patient's weight, relative to their height. The BMI is used as an indication of how underweight or overweight a patient is, and is determined by dividing body weight, in kg, by the square of the height in metres.

The BMI for a "normal" weight is said to be between 18.5 and 25, with obesity occurring at values of 30 or more.

📑 *Example 1*

Determine the BMI for a patient who weighs 68 kg, and has a height of 5 feet 5 inches.

◄◄◄ Solution ►►►

- ◆ Convert the 65 inch (5' 5") height from imperial to metric: 65 * 2.5 = 162.5 cm = 1.625 m.

- ◆ Square the height: 1.625 * 1.625 = 2.64.

◆ 68/2.64 = 25.75

Answer: BMI = 25.75

☑ *Example 2*

Determine the BMI for a patient who weighs 72 kg, and has a height of 1.8 metre.

◄◄◄ Solution ►►►

◆ Square the height: 1.8 * 1.8 = 3.24

◆ 72/3.24 = 22.22

Answer: BMI = 22.22

☆　☆　☆　☆　☆　☆　☆　☆　☆

Body Surface Area

Body Mass Index is not such a good indicator of the dosage requirements for some patients, such as in cardiac and paediatric cases so, instead, the *Body Surface Area* (m^2) is used.

In those environments where BSA is commonly used, calculations can be avoided, and a graphical system used instead. The graphical system, called a *Nomogram*, is implemented by means of connecting a patient's weight and height, from linear scales, and finding the BSA at an intersection point on a third linear scale.

Where a nomogram is unavailable, a calculation must be performed, using one of a variety of methods, with a popular method being the *Mosteller Formula*, where the product of height (cm) and weight (kg) is divided by 3,600, and the BSA determined by taking the square root of that calculation.

Square root of { [weight * height] / 3,600 }

📝 *Example*

Determine the BSA of a patient whose weight is 9.2 kg, and height is 45 cm.

◄◄◄ Solution ►►►

- ◆ Weight (9.2) * height (45) = 414.

- ◆ 414/3,600 = 0.115

- ◆ Square root of 0.115 = 0.339

Answer: Body Surface Area = 0.34 m² (rounded).

Note: In calculation tests, it would be usual to expect either a nomogram to be supplied, or a formula given. For more stringent tests, the formula may have to be used; which is why it is beneficial to become familiar with working with a given formula.

Tablet Dosages

The administration of oral medications, such as tablets and capsules, is a very popular and easy method of delivering drugs to patients, but the ease of administration makes the possibility of delivering an overdose very real.

The tablet dosage formula is a simple one; it is the prescribed dose divided by the supplied (stock) amount:

Number of tablets = Prescribed/supply

which can be remembered in a number of alternate ways, such as *what you want / what you have.*

To solve tablet dosage problems, the above fraction must be memorised. However, it is easy to forget which value is the numerator (top line), and which is the denominator (bottom line). A strategy is necessary, therefore, to obviate the need to trust in that most unreliable creature – memory.

One such strategy is to write down the basic facts about a prescription, before performing the calculation, necessary to meet the prescription instruction. Those basic facts are:

◆ Prescribed dose: larger font, if prescribed > supply.

◆ Supplied dose: larger font, if supply > prescribed.

◆ The expected outcome wil be one of:

  • Less than 1 tablet
  • Exactly 1 tablet.
  • More than 1 tablet.

If the prescribed dose is exactly the supplied amount, then no calculation is necessary, because the patient has been prescribed 1 tablet. Only the other two situations require calculation.

Note: the ">" symbol is a standard mathematical operator, meaning greater than, which does sometimes appear in clinical notes, so its use, although inferior to writing out **greater than**, is included here, to aid in gaining familiarity with it. Similarly, "<" is the standard operator to mean **less than**.

After completing the calculation, a quick check that the answer satisfies the above expected result, where the larger font is used to emphasise what is expected (less than OR greater than 1 tablet), helps to indicate that the calculation formula was used correctly (numerator and denominator correctly placed), and the prescribed dose was divided by the supplied amount - not the other way around.

For example, given the task of determining how many tablets are necessary to satisfy a prescribed dosage of 300 mg, using a supply of tablets which each contain 50 mg, the expected outcome would be declared in the following manner:

Prescribed = 300 mg

Supply = 50 mg.

*Expected answer is > (**more**) than one tablet.*

By writing the above prescribed value in a larger font than the supply value, it makes it obvious that the calculated answer should produce more than tablet, and the only way that type of answer can occur will be if the 300 (numerator) is divided by the 50 (denominator) i.e., 300/50, which gives **6** tablets. By checking the calculated answer with the previously declared "type" of answer expected (*more than 1 tablet*), we can be sure that the numerator and denominator were used the correct way around, specifically:

Prescribed dose

Supply dose

Conversely, if the problem is to administer, for example, 40 mg, using supply tablets of 120 mg, the declaration would be:

Prescribed = 40 mg

Supply = 120 mg.

*Expected answer is < (**less**) than one tablet.*

The above declaration shows that, because the prescribed dose (40) is smaller than the supply value, the calculated answer should be less than a whole tablet, and the only way that can occur is if the numerator is the smaller of the two values, which means 40 mg. The fraction formed is thus 40/120, which gives ⅓ of a tablet.

If you wrote the fraction with the numerator and denominator the wrong way around, your answer will not match your noted *expected answer* declaration which, in the above case, is ***less*** *than one tablet*. The action, in such a situation, would be to redo the calculation, with the fraction values reversed, thereby ensuring that the *Prescribed dose* (what you want) is on the top line (numerator) of the fraction. {*Alternatively, for those who are mathematically minded, correct the answer by taking the reciprocal.*}

📋 *Example 1*

A prescription for 750 mg drug D has been made, and the available supply (stock) is 300 mg tablets. How many tablets should be given?

◄◄◄ Solution ►►►

◆ The prescribed amount (750) is larger than the supplied amount (300), so the expected answer must be more than 1 tablet.

◆ Prescribed/supplied is 750/300 = 2.5

◆ The answer meets the expectation that more than 1 tablet is needed, therefore, the numerator / denominator are correct.

Answer: Prescribed/supply is 750/300 = 2.5 tablets.

📋 *Example 2*

A patient needs 8 g of drug E, supplied in tablets of 24 g each. How many tablets are required?

◄◄◄ Solution ►►►

◆ Prescribed amount is smaller than the supply, so the expected answer will be **less** than 1 tablet.

◆ Prescribed/supply is 8/24 = 0.33 (1/3) tablet.

◆ The answer meets the above expectation that the answer is **less** than one tablet, numerator / denominator are correct.

Answer: 0.33 tablet.

Ampoule/Bag Dosages

The above calculation principles, for tablet dosages, can be readily transposed to drugs supplied in bags, ampoules, and vials. The terminology of **prescribed dose** and **supply** amount stay the same.

✍ *Example 1*

A prescription reads 0.4 mg drug S, from supplied 250 microgram/5 ml ampoules. What volume should be drawn up?

◄◄◄ Solution ►►►

◆ Convert 0.4 mg to 400 microgram.

◆ Supply of 250/5 ml means 50 microgram/ml.

◆ The **prescribed** 400 microgram is larger than the 50 microgram/ml supply, so the expected answer must produce **more** than 1 ml.

◆ Prescribed/supply is 400/50 ≈ 8 ml.

◆ Each ampoule contains 5 ml, so 8/5 = 1.6 ampoules are needed.

Note: this satisfies the above expected answer: **more** *than 1 ampoule.*

Answer: 8 ml from 1.6 ampoules.

📋 *Example 2*

An order is for 2.5 million units of drug P, from a supply of ampoules containing 12 million unit/3 ml each. What volume should be prepared?

◄◄◄ Solution ►►►

◆ 12 million unit in 3 ml means 4 million per ml.

◆ The prescribed 2.5 million is smaller than the **supply** 4 million/ml supply, so the expected answer must be < 1 ampoule and < 1 ml.

◆ Prescribed/supply is 2.5/4 million = 0.625 ml, which matches the expected answer of less than 1 ampoule.

Answer: 0.6 ml (rounded).

📝 *Example 3*

If a patient must be given 150 microgram of a particular agent, and the agent is supplied in a suspension of 0.03 mg/ml, what volume of the supply should be prepared?

◄◄◄ Solution ►►►

◆ First, convert to common units: the supplied 0.03 mg * 1,000 = 30 microgram/ml.

◆ The **prescribed** dose (150 microgram) is larger than the supply (30 microgram/ml), therefore the expected answer is **greater** than 1 ml.

◆ Prescribed/supply is 150/30 = 5 ml.

Answer: 5 ml.

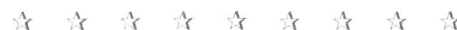

Drip Rates

A patient may be subject to intravenous infusion of a fluid which must be administered at an appropriate rate, governed by various factors, such as gravity, the difference in pressure between the fluid supply and the end of the tubing, the viscosity of the fluid, the length and bore of the tubing, and the setting of the flow controller (wheel).

The parameters (value types) needed, to complete a drip rate problem, include the following:

V: Total fluid volume to infuse

G: Giving set drip rate per ml (gtt)

R: Drops per minute/hour

T: Total administration time, minutes/hours

When tackling a drip rate problem, all but one of the given parameters will be given, and that missing value can be found by using the following formula:

Drip Rate Formula

V (volume) * **G** (drips/ml) = **R** (Drip rate) * **T** (time)

Which abbreviates to:

V * **G** = **R** * **T**

To find the missing value, simply divide both sides of the equation by its sibling; for example, if V (solution volume) is the unknown value, divide both sides by G, to give:

V = **R** * **T** / **G**

✎ *Example 1*

A patient is to receive 1 litre of fluid X, over 4 hours, using a giving set with a gtt (drops) per ml of 20. What rate, in drops/minute, should be set?

◄◄◄ Solution ►►►

Step 1: Convert to millilitres and minutes...

  V (solution volume) = 1,000 ml; T (time) = 240 mins.

Step 2: Declare the drip rate formula...

  VG = RT

Step 3: Rearrange to isolate the unknown parameter - R.

VG / T = R

Step 4: Calculate for R...

1,000 * 20 / 240 = R (drips/ml) = 83.3

Answer: 83 drops/minute.

◳ *Example 2*

A patient is prescribed an intravenous infusion, to be given over 4 hours, at a rate of 40 drops per minute, using a giving set with a gtt (drops/ml) of 15. What is the total amount of fluid which will be delivered?

◄◄◄ Solution ►►►

In this question, the answer is given differently from the above example – for variety.

Step 1: State the parameter values...

V = ?

G = 15

R = 40 drops/min

T = 240 minutes

Step 2:   Arrange the formula with V on one side…

   V = RT / G

Step 3: Solve V…

   V = 40 * 240 / 15 = 640

  Answer: 640 ml.

Pumped Infusions

When a more precise volume and infusion rate are needed, compared with that provided from a gravity type giving set, a pumped regime is required.

In this chapter, the simplest type of pumped infusion problem is described. *For more complex types of problem, refer to my other book –* **Pass Your Drug Calculation Test** *(Amazon Publishing).*

The infusion calculation is similar to that for tablets or ampoules, with the specific parameters for a flow rate per minute calculation being:

- ♣ Total volume to infuse.
- ♣ Infusion time.
- ♣ Infusion rate.

The precise relationship of the above parameters can be given by:

*Total volume infused = rate (ml/minute) * 60 * hours*

OR

Rate (ml/minute) = Total volume / Infusion time

Alternatively, follow these easy steps...

✎ *Example 1*

An infusion pump must be set to deliver a dose of 450 ml of fluid over 5 hours. What rate, per minute, should the pump be set to?

◄◄◄ Solution ►►►

- ◆ In 5 hours, 450 ml will be delivered.

- ◆ In 1 hour, 450/5 = 90 ml will be delivered.

- ◆ In 1 minute, 90/60 = 1.5 ml will be delivered.

Answer: 1.5 ml/min.

✎ *Example 2*

If 1 litre is to be infused at a rate of 4 ml/min, how long will it take to deliver the whole litre?

◄◄◄ Solution ►►►

If the delivery rate is 4 ml/min, then 1,000 ml will be delivered in 1,000/4 = 250 min.

Answer: 1 litre infused in 4 hours and 10 minutes.

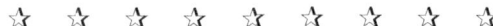

Displacement Volume

Definition

A specific volume of fluid is displaced when an object is placed into a particular space.

This can be easily exemplified by what happens when you take a bath, and note the water level before and after stepping in. The volume of water, which occupies the area between the "before" and "after" levels, is the volume which has been displaced by YOUR body, i.e., it is your *displacement volume* (Archimedes Principle).

In pharmacology, displacement volume is that which is occupied by a powdered drug, when reconstituted with a solvent. For example, if drug Q has a displacement volume of 0.1 ml/50 mg, and 250 mg in 10 ml is to be prepared, then only 9.5 ml of solvent must be added, because the remaining 0.5 ml is the volume displaced by the drug.

📝 Example 1

Calculate the volume of solvent required to produce 1 ml of a 5 mg solution of drug D, the displacement of which is 0.01 ml/mg.

◄◄◄ Solution ►►►

The given displacement volume of drug D is 0.01 ml per mg so, for 5 mg, the displacement volume is 0.05 ml.

To make up the 5 mg in 1 ml, 1 − 0.05 = 0.95 ml is required.

Answer: 0.95 ml.

📝 Example 2

Drug P, which has a displacement volume 0.56 ml/g, is to be prepared as a 4 ml solution of a 250 mg/ml concentration. How much water should be used to reconstitute drug P?

◄◄◄ Solution ►►►

To produce 4 ml of drug P, 1 g (4 * 250 mg) is needed. The given displacement volume is 0.56 ml per gram, so 4 − 0.56 = 3.44 ml solvent should be used to reconstitute drug P.

Answer: 3.44 ml.

To remember the principle on which a displacement volume calculation stands, simply recall the above described principle of the rising bath water level (*Archimedes principle)*: In the same way that YOUR immersion in a vessel (bath) displaces the water level, a powdered drug displaces the solvent in which it is immersed. The question to answer is – by how much (ml) does the immersed solute (drug) displace the solvent; in other words, what is the **displacement volume**?

Drug Concentration

Definition

In pharmacology, concentration describes the ratio of the amount of a drug to the solution in which it is contained.

The concentration can occur in several forms, such as:

♦ Molarity (M), which means the amount of the drug, in moles, per litre of solution. For example, 40 mmol (solute) in 100 ml (solution), has a molarity of 0.4, because 40 mmol in 100 ml is the same concentration as (* 10) 400 mmol in 1 litre.

♦ Mass to mass; more typically described as w/w (weight to weight). For example, 4 mg in 5 mg = 0.8.

♦ Volume to volume (v/v), such as 20 ml drug B in 500 ml normal saline = 4%.

♦ Mass to volume (density), or **weight to volume**,

also known as *mass concentration*, which describes how much solute a solution contains. For example, 100 mg in 1 ml has a concentration of 10%.

To understand pharmacological concentrations, it is useful, firstly, to consider the analogy of coffee "strength", where the amount of instant coffee, placed in a cup of a specific volume, determines how palatable the coffee will be; too much or too little coffee will be unpleasant to drink, whereas the right amount will be "just right". (The "right amount", in technical terms, means the right *weight/volume* concentration, as described above.)

With respect to pharmacological agents, the same situation exists: too little solvent, for a particular dose of the agent, will make the dose too concentrated (too strong), which could result, for example, in an unwanted reaction; too much solvent, clearly, will have the opposite effect – it will make the solution too "weak" to produce the desired clinical effect.

Rationale

Understanding the concentration of a drug is essential, because it describes the "strength" of agent being supplied. If the supplied drug is too "strong" (high concentration) to be administered to the patient, it must be weakened, by dilution, just as with the coffee example, which means decreasing the ratio of solute (drug) to solvent, by adding more of the solvent, such as saline, dextrose, or WFI (water for injections).

The ability to dilute (reduce) the concentration of a pharmacological agent is a mandatory skill for anyone administering, checking, or preparing drugs because, in most instances, a drug will be supplied in a higher concentration than is needed, because it allows the drug to be supplied in a smaller package. Consequently, a drug supplied in a higher than needed concentration requires less storage space than would be otherwise, and less space is a positive factor in resource utilisation (storage space costs money).

Note 1: Most pharmacological agents are supplied in amounts in terms of the previously mentioned mass of solute to volume of solution, described as the weight to volume (w/v) concentration, and this is the method described in this text.

Note 2: The term "weight", in the context of concentrations, is used synonymously, albeit incorrectly, with "mass" but, because "weight" is the everyday term to describe mass, that is (probably) why it is used within the realm of pharmacology – everyone is familiar with the concept of weight, so that is why it is used, instead of mass.

<u>Note 3:</u> To keep things simple, the issue of displacement volume will be ignored, and the volume of solution will be considered synonymous with volume of solvent.

Weight/Volume Concentration

The following text expands upon the previously defined weight/volume method, and the explanations and examples, therein, should be studied and re-studied, until this subject is mastered, not only because it is essential for patient safety, but also because it helps to understand more advanced types of describing drug concentrations, particularly *molarity*, which is the most important and fundamental measurement system in pharmacology.

Weight/Volume Reference Values

Before calculating a weight/volume concentration problem, it is necessary to understand what the concentration value, as a percentage, means. Quite simply, if 1 g of a substance is dissolved in a solution of 1 ml volume, then the concentration of solute to solution is described as **1 in 1, or 100%**.

Most texts use the fact that 1 g of a solute (drug) in 100 ml of solution means a w/v concentration of 1%, and use this fact as a reference value, from which other concentrations may be derived. The problem with this approach is that most drug concentrations, in ampoules and storage packets, are described as being a certain mass of solute in 1 ml of solution – not 100 ml; for example, 10 mg in 1 ml. So, using 100 ml as a reference value is, arguably, a counter-intuitive model for using a reference value.

A better approach is to remember that 10 mg (one hundredth of 1 gram), in 1 ml of solution, is a 1% concentration. This is particularly relevant because many drugs are supplied in these 1% solutions. For example, Lidocaine, Morphine, and Propofol. A look at the packaging or labels of any of these drugs will confirm this fact and, by doing so, serves to encourage a more easily remembered reference value, namely, 10 mg/ml is a w/v concentration of 1%.

⬛ *Weight/Volume Example 1*

Convert a 3 mg/ml solution to a w/v concentration.

◄◄◄ Solution ►►►

♦ Using the 1% Lidocaine reference value, where a 1% w/v concentration means *10 mg/ml*, comparing 3 mg as a fraction of 10 mg, gives 3/10, or 0.33.

♦ 3 mg/ml w/v is 0.33 of the 1% w/v concentration of the 10 mg reference solution, which is **0.33%**.

Answer: 0.33% w/v.

⬛ *Weight/Volume Example 2*

What is the w/v concentration of a 200 microgram in 5 ml solution?

◄◄◄ Solution ►►►

Before completing the calculation, simplify the given 200 microgram/5 ml solution to a 1 ml concentration, which is 40 microgram in 1 ml.

The 40 microgram value is much smaller than the 10 mg/ml (1%) reference value, so the w/v value must also be smaller, and this fact serves as a useful check of the calculation. To determine the 40 microgram/ml concentration, note down successively smaller concentrations, until the target (40 microgram) concentration is found, by dividing each time (as if diluting) subsequent concentrations by 10:

Solution	W/V concentration
10 mg/ml	1 in 100 (1%)
1 mg/ml	1 in 1,000
100 microgram/ml	1 in 10,000
10 microgram/ml	1 in 100,000

From the above list, 40 microgram/ml is 4 times the amount in 10 microgram/ml, therefore, 40 microgram/ml is 4 in 100,000.

Answer: 4 in 100,000, or 1 in 25,000

In summary

The concept of a drug concentration is not as complicated as it may at first appear, and the strategy for solving the most commonly encountered concentration problem, weight/volume, can be reliably based on remembering the reference value of a commonly available agent with a 1% weight/volume concentration (10 mg/ml), such as 1% Lidocaine.

W/V Concentration – Method 2

For the reader who is comfortable with using basic equations, weight/volume problems can be solved by a formulaic method, using the following canonical (main) equation:

mass (g) = concentration * solution volume (ml)

All of the w/v problem parameters are collated in the above equation and, by simple manipulation, any of the unknown values can be determined.

📝 *Example – Drug Mass?*

What mass of solute (drug) is there in 20 ml of a 3% solution?

◄◄◄ Solution ►►►

Step 1: Declare the formula...

drug mass (g) = w/v concentration * volume (ml)

Step 2: Convert % to decimal...

3% = 0.03

Step 3: Realize the parameters...

Drug (solute) mass = 0.03 * 20 g

Step 4: Resolve the equation...

Mass = 20 * 0.03 = 0.6 g = 600 mg

Answer: 600 mg.

If it is not the drug (solute) mass which is to be found, then one of the following formula derivations should be used:

Finding the Solution Volume

solution volume = mass/concentration

Example – Solution Volume?

What is the volume of a solution containing 10 mg of a 1

in 2,000 concentration?

◄◄◄ Solution ►►►

Step 1: Convert 1 in 2,000 to a decimal...

   1 / 2,000 = 0.0005

Step 2: Convert 10 mg to g...

   10/1,000 = 0.01 g

Step 3: Use the formula...

   Volume = 0.01 / 0.0005 = 20 ml

Answer: 20 ml.

Finding the W/V Concentration

concentration = drug mass (g) / volume (ml)

✎ *Example – W/V?*

What is the w/v concentration of 200 microgram (solute) in a 10 ml solution?

◄◄◄ Solution ►►►

Step 1: Convert to microgram to g...

  200 microgram = 0.0002 g

Step 2: Declare the formula...

  w/v concentration = drug mass (g) / volume (ml)

Step 3: Realize the parameters...

  W/V = 0.0002 / 10 = 0.00002 (0.002%)

Answer: 1 in 50,000 (or 0.002%).

☆ ☆ ☆ ☆ ☆ ☆ ☆ ☆ ☆

Dilutions

Definition

The concept of *dilution* is something which is instinctive, and part of normal life experience for most people.

For example, using the previously described analogy of coffee, if it is too "strong", the natural reaction would be to make the drink "weaker", by reducing the amount of coffee (solute) relative to the water (solvent) or, in other words, changing the *weight/volume* concentration.

This process of diluting a product, which even small children understand, is, in chemistry terms, a process of concentration reduction, and most people understand this basic concept of chemistry, even though they may not realise it themselves!

Pharmacological Dilutions

When a drug has to be diluted, the correct type of of solvent, which provides the diluent, must be used, usually according to supplier instructions. The type of solvent to use will, typically, be one of: Dextrose, WFI (Water For Injections), or Normal (0.9%) Saline.

> <u>Note</u>:   In some instances, the choice of solvent is specific to one particular type, and in other instances there may be a choice of two or more solvents. Supplier instructions, or local policies, determine the solvents to use, and these instructions should be regarded as part of the proper administration regime.

☑ *Dilution Example 1*

Drug E is supplied as 1 ml of a 3% w/v concentration, and must be diluted to 3 mg/ml. How should the final solution be composed?

◄◄◄ Solution ►►►

♦   Firstly: note that our chosen reference value of 1% Lidocaine has a concentration of 10 mg/ml.

♦ Secondly: the supplied solution of 3%, is 3 times the concentration of the reference value of 1% and, therefore, has 3 times the mass in the same volume, i.e., 3 * 10 mg = 30 mg in 1 ml.

♦ Thirdly: the task is to reduce the supplied 30 mg/ml to just 3 mg/ml, which means either drawing up one tenth (3/30) of the supplied drug and making up the 1 ml with solvent/diluent, or (preferred method) drawing up all of the supplied drug, then making it up to 10 ml by adding solvent/diluent, producing 30 mg in 10 ml (3 mg/ml).

Method 1: Draw up 0.1 ml (3 mg) of the supplied ampoule into a 1 ml syringe, then add 0.9 ml of diluent to produce the full 1 ml. The resultant solution will be **3 mg in 1 ml**. (*Note: this method is only valid if just 1 ml of 3 mg/ml is needed. If more than 1 ml is required, method 2 is the appropriate option.*)

Method 2: Draw up all of the ampoule's 30 mg (1 ml) into a 10 ml syringe, and add a further 9 ml of diluent, to produce a concentration of 30 mg in 10 ml, which resolves to the required **3 mg/ml**.

☞ *Dilution Example 2*

Drug K is supplied as 2 ml of a 5% w/v, and must be used to create 3 ml of a 10 mg/ml concentration. How can this be achieved?

◄◄◄ Solution, method 1 ►►►

◆ Producing 3 ml of 10 mg/ml means **30 mg in 3 ml**.

◆ Note: 1% w/v is 10 mg/ml.

◆ 5% w/v is 5 * 10 mg/ml = 50 mg/ml.

◆ Extract 30 mg from 50 mg/ml: draw up 3/5 = 0.6 ml.

◆ Add 3 - 0.6 = 2.4 ml of diluent, gives 30 mg in 3 ml.

Answer: 2.4 ml diluent + 0.6 ml of the 5% concentration of drug K.

◄◄◄ Method 2 ►►►

◆ Add 3 ml saline to the 2 ml of 5%, giving 100 mg in 5 ml, or 20 mg/ml, which is 2% w/v.

◆ Extract 1.5 ml to give 30 mg in 1.5 ml.

◆ Add 1.5 ml saline to give 30 mg in 3 ml, which is 10 mg/ml.

Calculation Test

The following questions represent what could be found in a drug calculation test, and which might be considered to be of a minimum standard.

With persistence and regular practice, and with frequency determined by individual needs, even the most numerically weak practitioners should develop the skills necessary to master the types of calculation included in this selection of drug dosage problems. So, practice, practice, practice.

Questions & Answers

Q 1. The SI unit for the amount of something is:

a. The Newton

b. The Mole

c. The Kilogram

Answer: b, the Mole.

Q 2. The SI unit for volume is the litre; True or false?

False. The litre is an SI *derived* unit.

Q 3. The SI unit for weight is:

w. The Kilogram

x. The Newton

y. The Gram

z. There is no SI unit for weight.

Answer: z. Gram and Kilogram are mass, and the Newton is an SI derived unit for weight.

Q 4. The SI unit for temperature is Celsius; True or false?

False. SI temperature units are in the Kelvin scale.

Q 5. Convert 0.0055 g to micrograms.

A gram is one million times the value of a microgram, so multiplying 0.0055 by a million gives

Answer: 5,500 microgram.

Q 6. Convert 27,495 microgram to mg.

Each 1,000 microgram is one mg, so, divide by 1,000.

Answer: 27.495 mg.

Q 7. How many milligrams are there in 0.04 gram?

One thousand milligrams comprise one gram, so multiplying 0.04 g by a thousand gives:

Answer: 40 mg.

Q 8. There are 10,000 nanograms in one milligram; True or false?

Answer: False; One million nanogram = 1 mg.

Q 9. Convert 0.55 litre to ml.

One litre contains 1,000 ml, so 0.55 litre contains 1,000 * 0.55 = 550 ml.

Answer: 550 ml.

Q 10. Convert 1,200 micromoles to moles.

◆ <u>Note a</u>: 1,000 micromol = 1 mmol.

◆ <u>Note b</u>: 1,000 mmol = 1 mol.

◆ 1,200 micromol / 1,000 = 1.2 millimol.

◆ 1.2 millimol / 1,000 = 0.0012 mol.

Answer: 0.0012 mol.

Q 11. A patient, who weighs 66 kg, has been prescribed a dose of drug B, which should be measured as 6 mg per kg of body weight. How much should be given?

Answer: 66 * 6 = 396 mg.

Q 12. A patient, who weighs 72 kg, needs a regime of a medication which is dosed at 15 mg/kg/6 hour. What is the total daily dose?

Each dose is 15 * 72 = 1,080 mg. The daily dose is 4 * 1,080 = 4,320 mg = 4.32 g.

Answer: 4.32 g.

Q 13.   Calculate the Body Mass Index for a patient whose weight is 110 kg, and height is 5 feet 10 inches.

◆ Write down the formula for BMI:

Weight / (height*height), using kg/m^2.

◆ Convert 5 feet 10 inch to inches: (5 * 12) + 10 = 70 inch.

◆ Convert 70 inch to cm. 70 * 2.5 = 175 cm.

◆ Convert 175 cm to metres: 175/100 = 1.75 m.

◆ Square the height: 1.75 * 1.75 = 3.0625 m^2.

◆ Use the BMI formula: 110/3.0625 = 35.92.

Answer: BMI is 35.9.

Q 14. Calculate the BMI for a patient whose weight is 64 kg, and height is 150 cm.

◆ Write down the formula for BMI:

Weight / (height*height), using kg/m^2.

◆ Convert 150 cm to metres: 150/100 = 1.5 m.

◆ Create the square of the height: 1.5 * 1.5 = 2.25 m^2.

◆ Use the BMI formula: 64/2.25 = 28.4.

Answer: BMI is 28.4.

Q 15. What is the Body Surface Area of a 80 cm child who weighs 25 kg?

◆ Recall the BSA formula:

*Square root of { [body weight * height] / 3600}*, where weight is in kg, and height is in cm.

◆ Weight * height = 25 * 80 cm = 2,000.

◆ 2,000/3,600 = 0.55

◆ Square root of 0.55 = 0.74

Answer: BSA = 0.74 m².

Q 16. A preparation of drug Q, at 120 microgram per square metre of body area, is required for a patient who weighs 15 kg, and height 55 cm. Drug Q is supplied in ampoules with concentration of 50 microgram/ml. How much drug X should be drawn up?

◆ Declare the BSA formula:

*Square root of { [body weight * height] / 3600}.*

◆ Weight * height = 15 * 55 = 825.

◆ 825/3,600 = 0.23.

◆ BSA is the square root of 0.23 = 0.478 m².

◆ Dose is 0.478 * 120 microgram = 57.36 microgram.

Answer: 1.15 ml.

Q 17. A patient, who weighs 84 kg, is prescribed drug Z, 80 microgram/kg/3 times a day, which is supplied in ampoules of 10 mg/5 ml. What is the total daily volume required?

◆ A single dose is 84 * 80 = 6,720 microgram = 6.72 mg.

◆ The daily dose is 6.72 * 3 = 20.16 mg.

◆ **Prescribed** (20.16 mg) is > **(greater** than) the supply (10 mg); expected answer is > 1 ampoule.

◆ Ampoules required: 20.16 mg/10 mg = 2.016 (as expected).

◆ Each supplied ampoule contains 5 ml, so the volume needed is 2.016 * 5 = 10.08 ml.

Answer: 10.1 ml (rounded up).

Q 18. Calculate the volume of solvent (0.9% saline) required to produce 2 ml of a 10 mg solution of drug D, the displacement of which is 0.08 ml/5 mg.

◆ Displacement volume of drug D is 0.08 ml per 5 mg.

◆ 10 mg are prescribed, so 10/5 = 2 times the 0.08 ml displacement amount will exist, i.e., 0.16 ml.

◆ To make up the volume to 2 ml, the 2 – 0.16 = 1.84 ml of solvent is required.

Answer: 1.84 ml solvent.

Q 19. Drug P, which has a displacement volume 0.56 ml/g, is to be prepared as a 4 ml solution of a 250 mg/ml concentration. How much solvent should be used to reconstitute drug P?

◆ To produce 4 ml of drug P, 4 * 250 mg = 1 g is needed.

◆ The displacement volume is 0.56 ml/g, so 4 – 0.56 = 3.44 ml solvent should be used to reconstitute drug P.

Answer: 3.44 ml.

Q 20. Drug P has a displacement volume of 0.5 ml per 20 mg. If 100 mg of drug P, in 20 ml WFI, should be prepared, how much WFI should be used to reconstitute the 100 mg of drug P?

◆ Displacement volume of 100 mg drug P is 100/20 = 5 times the displacement volume of the above 20 mg, which means 5 * 0.5 = 2.5 ml.

◆ Add to the 100 mg drug P: 20 – 2.5 = 17.5 ml WFI.

Answer: Reconstitute 100 mg drug P with 17.5 ml WFI.

Q 21. A 600 mg prescription for an IV dose of drug G is made, and drug G is supplied in ampoules of 250 mg/10 ml. How much (ml) should be drawn up?

◆ **Prescribed** (600 mg) > supplied ampoule (250 mg), so expected answer is **more** than 1 ampoule.

◆ The number of ampoules needed is calculated from the *prescribed dose / supply amount*, which is 600/250 = 12/5 = 2.4 ampoules. *(This meets the above check.)*

◆ Each ampoule contains a 10 ml solution, so 2.4 ampoules contains 2.4 * 10 = 24 ml.

Answer: 24 ml.

Q 22. If a patient is prescribed 1.5 g of drug P, which is supplied in 125 mg tablets, how many tablets are required?

◆ First, convert to a common unit: 1.5 g is 1,500 mg.

◆ (**Prescribed**) **1,500** > 125 mg; expected answer is > 1 tablet.

◆ Second, translate prescribed/supply into 1,500/125 mg = 12, which meets expected answer.

Answer: 12 tablets.

Q 23. The patient is prescribed 150 microgram of drug R, which is supplied in 300 microgram tablets, how many tablets are required?

◆ Prescribed (150 microgram) < (less than) **supply**

(300 microgram), so expected answer is **less** than 1 tablet.

✦ Prescribed/supply is 150/300 = 0.5, which matches the expected answer.

Answer: 0.5 (half) of one tablet.

Q 24. A prescription of 750 mg is made for drug A, which is supplied in tablet form, containing 300 mg. How many tablets are needed?

✦ Prescribed (750 mg) > supply (300 mg), so expected answer is **more** than 1 tablet.

✦ Prescribed/supply is 750/300 = 2.5. (*Expected > 1*)

Answer: 2.5 tablets.

Q 25. A prescription states that the patient should be given an oral medication of 0.6 mg of drug B, 4 times a day. Drug B is supplied in tablets of 80 microgram each. How many tablets a day should the patient be given?

✦ Convert 0.6 mg to microgram = 600 microgram.

◆ Daily, 600 * 4 = 2,400 microgram.

◆ **2,400 (prescribed)** is > than 80 microgram (supply), so expected answer is **more** than 1 tablet.

◆ Daily dose of 2,400 microgram requires (prescribed/supply) 2,400/80 = 30 tablets, which matches the expected answer.

Answer: 30 tablets.

Q 26. The patient is prescribed 2.5 mg drug V, from a supply of 200 microgram/ml ampoules, each containing 5 ml. What volume should be drawn up?

◆ Convert 2.5 mg to 2,500 microgram.

◆ **2,500 (prescribed)** > 200 microgram, so expected answer is **more** than 1 ml.

◆ Prescribed/supply is 2,500/200 = 12.5 ml (expected).

Answer: 12.5 ml.

Q 27. If a patient is to be given 0.8 mg of drug X, with a total volume of 5 ml, what is the concentration of the supplied ampoules?

◆ Convert 0.8 mg to 0.8 * 1,000 = 800 microgram.

◆ 800 microgram in 5 ml is 800/5 = 160 microgram/ml.

Answer: 160 microgram/ml.

Q 28. The patient has been prescribed 900 mg of drug A, which is supplied in 1 ml ampoules, containing 250 mg. How many ampoules of drug F should be drawn up?

◆ **900 mg (prescribed)** > 250 mg(supply), so expected answer is **more** than 1 ampoule.

◆ The number of ampoules is given by 900/250 = 3.6 (Meets expected answer: > 1).

Answer: 3.6 ampoules.

Q 29. You have to prepare a solution with 300 mg of drug Q, which is supplied in bags of 500 mg in 200 ml. How much of the bag do you need?

◆ 300 mg (prescribed) < **500 mg (supply)**, so the expected answer is **less** than 1 bag.

◆ Prescribed/supply is 300/500 = 0.6 of a bag (expected). 0.6 of 200 = 120 ml.

Answer: 120 ml.

Q 30. You have the task of preparing a syringe of 270 mg of drug T, which is supplied as 60 mg/4 ml. How much should you draw up?

◆ 60 mg/4 ml is 15 mg/ml.

◆ **Prescribed (270 mg)** > supply (15 mg), so the answer will be **more** than 1 ml.

◆ Prescribed/Supply is 270/15 = 18 ml.

Answer: 18 ml.

Q 31. A prescription for a 20 mg IV bolus of drug F is to be realised, using a supplied ampoule containing 75 mg in 5 ml of solvent. How much drug F should be drawn up?

◆ Prescribed (20 mg) < **supply (75 mg)**, so expected answer is **less** than 1 ampoule.

◆ The ampoule contains 75/5 = 15 mg/ml.

◆ To deliver the prescribed dose: *prescribed/supply* is 20/15 = 1.33 ml.

Answer: 1.33 ml.

Q 32. If a patient is to be given a 150 unit infusion of drug J, which is supplied in 60 unit per 10 ml ampoules, how much drug J should be given?

◆ **150 unit (prescribed)** > 60 IU, so expected answer is more than 1 ampoule.

◆ Prescribed/supplied is 150/60 = 2.5 ampoules.

◆ Each ampoule contains 10 ml, so 2.5 ampoules gives 10 * 2.5 = 25 ml.

Answer: 25 ml.

Q 33. Drug M is supplied in ampoules of 500 mg in 8 ml. A patient, who weighs 35 kg, has been prescribed 3 mg/kg of drug M. What volume of drug M should be prepared?

♦ The required (prescribed) dose is 35 * 3 = 105 mg.

♦ Prescribed (105) < the **supply** (**500**) mg, so expected answer is **less** than 1 ampoule.

♦ The 105 mg must be taken from the supply of 500 mg in 8 ml, which is a fraction of an ampoule found by 105/500 = 0.21 ampoule.

♦ An ampoule contains 8 ml, so 0.21 ampoule is 0.21 * 8 = 1.68 ml. (It is reasonable to round up to 1.7 ml.)

Answer: 1.7 ml.

Q 34. If a patient is given a 3 L infusion of a fluid, via a standard giving set, over 5 hours, what is the administration rate, per minute?

In one hour, 3/5 L is given, which is 600 ml.

In one minute, 600/60 = 10 ml is given.

Answer: 10 ml per minute.

Q 35. How many drops per minute are administered, via a giving set having a gtt of 20 (20 drops/ml), if 1.2 L is infused over 3 hours? (Use the formula method)

◆ Drip rate formula: VG = RT

◆ Isolate the unknown parameter (R)...

  R = (VG) / T

◆ Use the given values...

  R = (1,200 ml * 20 drops/ml) / 180 minutes = 133.33

Answer: 133⅓ drops per minute.

Q 36. For an infusion regime of 2.5 L, via a giving set, over five hours, and at a rate of 125 drops/min, what is the gtt of the giving set? (Solved without the formula method)

◆ In one hour, 2.5/5 L = 500 ml is given.

◆ In terms of drops, 125 * 60 = 7,500 drops are given in one hour.

◆ Drops/ml is found by: 7,500 drops by 500 ml = 15.

Answer: gtt/ml is 15 drops per ml.

Q 37. The patient is to be given 750 ml over 3 hours, using a giving set with a gtt/ml of 15. How many drops/minute should be delivered?

♦ If 750 ml are delivered in 3 hours, then 750/3 = 250 ml will be delivered in 1 hour.

♦ Converting to drops, 250 * 15 = 3,750 drops in 1 hour.

♦ In 1 minute, 3,750 / 60 = 125/2 = 62.5 drops/minute.

Answer: 62.5 drops/min.

Q 38. An IV infusion of 1 litre, using a giving set with a gtt/ml of 20, must be administered over 4 hours. How many drops per minute should be set?

♦ To infuse 1,000 ml in 4 hours means 250 ml/hour.

♦ Converting to drops, 250 * 20 = 5,000 drops/hour.

♦ In one minute, 5,000/60 = 83.3 drops/minute.

Answer: 83 drops/min (rounded).

Q 39. An infusion pump must be set to deliver an IV dose of 500 ml of fluid over 4 hours. What rate, per minute, should the pump be set to?

In one hour, 500/4 = 125 ml must be delivered.

In one minute, 125/60 = 2.08 ml must be delivered.

Answer: 2.1 ml (rounded up).

Q 40. A patient is to be given 0.8 g of drug J over 5 hours. Drug J is supplied as bags of 1 g in 500 ml. Determine the infusion volume, per minute?

◆ Supply: 1,000/500 is **2 mg**/ml.

◆ Convert 0.8 g to mg: 0.8 * 1,000 = 800 mg/5 hours.

◆ In 1 hour, 800/5 = 160 mg will be infused.

◆ In 1 minute, 160/60 = **2.67 mg** should be infused.

◆ Prescribed/supply is 2.67/2 mg = 1.335 ml.

Answer: 1.34 ml/min (rounded).

Q 41. A patient is to be given 0.8 g of drug G over 10 hours. If drug G is delivered in a solution (bag) of 40 mg per 50 ml of solution, what rate, per hour, should the infusion pump be set to?

◆ Convert to common units; 0.8 g = 800 mg.

◆ 800 mg in 10 hours means 80 mg per hour.

◆ Each 40 mg is contained in 50 ml solution, so 80 mg must be in 80/40 = 2 bags of 50 ml.

◆ 2 * 50 = 100 ml.

Answer: Infusion rate of 100 ml/hour.

Q 42. A 5% w/v supply of drug D is served in a 250 ml solution. How much of drug D is this?

◆ Remembering that a 1% w/v concentration (reference value) means 10 mg/ml, a 5% concentration is 5 times the 1% value. So, 5% w/v means 5 * 10 = 50 mg/ml.

◆ As there are 250 ml of the 5% w/v concentration, then there is 250 * 50 = 12,500 mg, or 12.5 g, of drug D in the solution.

Answer: 12.5 g.

Q 43. Drug P is supplied in a w/v concentration of 4%. The patient requires 12 g of drug P. What volume of drug P is required?

◆   Convert 12 g to mg = 12,000 mg.

◆   The w/v concentration reference value, Lidocaine 1%, is 10 mg/ml. 4% w/v, therefore, means 4 * 10 = 40 mg/ml.

◆   To   deliver   (12,000   mg),   12,000/40 (*prescribed/supply*) = 300 ml.

Answer: 300 ml.

Q 44. A patient is subject to a 2.5 litre administration of an infusion of drug X, which has a w/v concentration of 15%. How much drug X is administered?

◆ A 1% w/v concentration (reference) means 10 mg/ml.

◆ 15% w/v means 10 mg * 15 = 150 mg/ml.

◆ For 2.5 litre, 150 mg * 2,500 = 375,000 mg.

◆ Convert to grams; 375,000 mg / 1,000 = 375 g.

Answer: 375 g.

Q 45. Drug T is supplied as 1 ml of a 2% w/v concentration, and must be diluted to 8 mg/ml. How should the final solution be composed?

<u>Note</u>: Before doing the calculation, it is helpful to use the coffee analogy which, in this case, means assuming a cup of coffee having 20 spoons of sugar must be diluted (less sweet) to effectively become a cup with only 8 spoons of sugar. Intuitively, everyone knows this type of dilution means having to add more solvent (water), until the required (8 sugars) sweetness is produced. To change the 20 mg/ml concentration of drug T to only 8 mg/ml means diluting, as with the coffee analogy, by adding a solvent.

◆ Note the reference value of 1% Lidocaine, which has a concentration of 10 mg/ml.

◆ 2% Drug T is double the above: 2 * 10 = 20 mg/ml.

◆ Drug T required is 8/20 = **0.4** of the supplied concentration; which is 8 mg in 0.4 ml.

◆ To create the 8 mg/ml concentration, add 0.6 ml of solvent.

Answer: Draw up 0.4 ml of drug T (supply), and add 0.6 ml solvent.

Q 46. Drug F is supplied as ampoules of 100 microgram in 2 ml. For a paediatric patient, the required dose is 20 microgram of a 10 microgram/ml concentration. How is this achieved?

◆ Draw up 50 microgram (1 ml) of drug F.

◆ Add 4 ml of solvent to the above 50 microgram, to produce 50 microgram/5 ml, or 10 microgram/ml.

◆ Draw up 2 ml of the 10 microgram/ml solution.

Answer: Administer 2 ml of the above 10 microgram/ml.

Q 47. A 20 ml solution of a 20% w/v concentration of drug A is to be drawn up. Only a 50% supply of drug A is available. How should the 20 ml of 20% be prepared?

The prescribed/supply fraction of 20/50 = 0.4 means only 0.4 of the required 20 ml is from the 50% supply, and the remaining 12 ml should be solvent.

Answer: Draw up 8 ml of the 50% supply, and add 12 ml solvent.

Q 48. 40 ml of a solution of drug M must be prepared, from a supply of 10 mg/ml ampoules, such that the solution produced is a 1 in 1,000 concentration. How should this be prepared?

◆ Firstly, determine the solution which satisfies the requirement that it has a 1 in 1,000 concentration: the easiest way to determine this is to utilise our knowledge (aide-memoire) that a 1% solution of, for example, Lidocaine, contains 10 mg/ml.

◆ With the above knowledge, it becomes easy to derive what a 1 in 1,000 solution means, because a 1 in 1,000 solution is one tenth the concentration of a 1% (1 in 100), and one tenth the concentration of 10 mg/ml is 1 mg/ml. The required concentration, therefore, is **1 mg/ml**.

◆ If 40 ml is required, then there will be 40 mg of drug M, and that amount can be found from 4 ampoules, because each ampoule contains 10 mg.

◆ Each ampoule contains 1 ml of solvent (0.9% saline), so the 40 mg is contained in 4 ml i.e., 40 mg/4 ml.

◆ To produce the desired concentration of 1 mg/ml, the above 4 ml solution must be made up to 40 ml by adding 36 ml of solvent, thus producing 40 mg/40 ml, which is, of course, a concentration of 1 mg/ml.

Answer: Add 36 ml normal saline to the combined 4 ampoules of drug M.

Q 49. To dilute a solution, add more solute; True or false?

Answer: False. That will increase the concentration. Dilution means adding more diluent.

Q 50. A solution of 1 mg in 1 ml means 1% w/v concentration; True or false?

Answer: False; 1 mg/ml is 1 in 1,000 (10 mg/ml); 1% means 10 mg/ml.

☆ ☆ ☆ ☆ ☆ ☆ ☆ ☆ ☆

Student Sample Questions

The following six questions are part of drug calculation tests, posted on Twitter, by student nurses who asked for help with the solutions. Note: question 2 might be considered intermediate rather than a basic level question.

(1) A patient is accidentally given 10,000 units more heparin than prescribed. Immediately following the dose, the antagonist protamine (1% w/v) must be given, at 1 mg for every 100 units of heparin. How much protamine should be given?

A w/v of 1% means 10 mg/ml protamine.

Each 100 units heparin needs 1 mg protamine, so 10,000/100 = 100 mg protamine is needed.

Volume of protamine needed is 100/10 = 10 ml.

Answer: 10 ml of 1% protamine.

(2) A patient needs an infusion of dobutamine, at a rate of 2 microgram/kg/min. The patient weighs 50 kg. The supply is 200 mg in 500 ml glucose 5% solution. What is the rate in ml/hour?

Convert to microgram:

200 mg = 200,000 microgram.

Equation for pumped infusions is:

$$m * r = d * w * f$$

drug mass * rate = dose * patient weight * fluid

Isolate the unknown variable "r":

rate = dose * patient weight * fluid / drug mass

r   = d * w * f / m

Substituting values into the variables:

r = 2 * 50 * 500 / 200,000 = 0.25 ml/minute

0.25 ml/minute * 60 = 15 ml/hour.

Answer: 15 ml/hour.

(3) A patient has chest pain, and is prescribed a glyceryltrinitrate (GTN) infusion, at a rate of 10 microgram/minute. Using a 50 mg in 50 ml supply, what is the infusion volume per hour?

* An infusion rate of 10 microgram/minute means 600 microgram/hour (10 * 60).

* The 50 mg/50 ml supply means 1 mg/ml.

* 1 mg is 1,000 microgram, so 600 microgram can be found in 0.6 (600/1,000) ml.

Answer: 0.6 ml/hour.

(4) A 800 mg dose of dopamine, in a 250 ml solution of D5W, must be infused at 10 microgram/kg/minute, for a patient who weighs 85 kg. What is the rate/hour?

* Convert the given dose regime to per hour: 10 * 60 = 600 microgram/kg/hour.

* Convert to mg: 600 microgram = 0.6 mg/hour.

* Hourly mg is 85 * 0.6 = 51 mg/hour.

* 51 mg is a 51/800 = 0.06375 fraction of the 250 ml.

* 0.06375 * 250 = 15.9 ml/hour.

Answer: 16 ml/hour (rounded).

(5) Using normal saline and 10 ml of 0.5% w/v bupivacaine, how would you make up a 5 ml solution of 0.375% w/v bupivacaine?

* Note that 1% w/v means 10 mg/ml.

* The 0.375% solution is a 0.375/1 fraction of 10 mg, which is 3.75 mg/ml.

* A 5 ml solution is 5 * 3.75 = 18.75 mg.

* The supplied 0.5% solution means 5 mg/ml.

* To get the required 18.75 mg, how many ml of the 0.5% solution are required?

* It takes 18.75/5 = 3.75 ml of the 0.5% supply to give the 18.75 mg needed, and so the remaining 1.25 ml must come from the normal saline.

Answer: Add 1.25 ml saline to 3.75 ml of the supplied 0.5% bupivacaine.

(6) Given a 200 ml supply of 2.5% w/v drug X, what is the weight (mass) of the supplied drug X?

* Using the standard 1% lidocaine as a reference, where 1% w/v means 10 mg/ml, 2.5% must be 10 mg * 2.5, which is 25 mg/ml.

* The supply is 200 ml of 2.5%, so there must be 200 * 25 mg in total i.e., 5,000 mg, or 5 g.

Answer: 5 g drug X.

Glossary & Abbreviations

In terms of safety, using abbreviations to describe drug dosage factors introduces an increased probability of making errors and, therefore, produces increased risk to patients.

Dosage abbreviations are, unfortunately, still used, to some degree, but their use is best avoided, particularly Latin abbreviations unless, of course, everyone speaks Latin! For completeness, some example abbreviations are included in the following list of terms.

AC: Before food.

Ampoule: A sealed glass or plastic container for fluid.

BD/BID: Twice daily.

BIS: Twice.

Body Mass Index: A numerical value, calculated from a patient's mass and height, which indicates whether the patient is relatively under or over weight.

Body Surface Area: The area of the external surface of the body.

Buccal: The mouth/cheek.

Concentration: The description of how closely packed things are, or the density of particles in their containing medium.

Cubic centimetre (USA: centimeter): The volume described by a cube of 1 cm sides; equivalent to one millilitre.

D5W: A solution of 5% w/v dextrose in water.

D10W: A solution of 10% w/v dextrose in water.

Dilution: The product of reducing the concentration of a solution, by adding more solvent.

Displacement volume: The volume of fluid which is displaced when an object is immersed in it.

Drip rate: The amount of fluid, measured in drops/second, ejected from a giving set.

Drop factor: See GTT.

Formulary: A list of drug descriptions and administration rules.

GTT: The number of drops which constitute one ml of liquid, delivered by a giving set.

ID: Intradermal.

IM: Intramuscular.

IV: Intravenous.

Nomogram: Graphical scales which allow a derived value to be found from the intersection of two other scales.

Normal Saline: Salt water with a salinity giving a tonicity which matches the tonicity (0.89%) of human tissue and cellular fluid.

OD: Every day.

PO: Orally.

PR: By rectum.

PRN: When needed.

QD: Once a day.

QDS: Four times a day.

QQH: Every four hours.

SI: *Système International d'Unités* - The canonical set of measurement systems, from which other systems are derived.

Solute: That part of a solution which has been dissolved by a solvent.

Solution: The product of dissolving a solute into a solvent.

Solvent: That part of a solution in which a solute dissolves.

Speed Shock: Sudden reaction to an intravenous drug that has been administered too quickly

Stat: Immediately.

Subq: Subcutaneous.

TDS/**TID**: Three times a day.

TPN: Total parenteral nutrition.

Unit: An International Unit is the amount of a particular agent that produces a specific biological effect.

V/V: The relative volumes of one fluid to another fluid.

W/V: The relative weight of one substance to the volume of another.

W/W: The relative weights of one substance to another.

WFI: Water For Injections.

Books by John England

📖 **Glossary of Anaesthetics**
http://amzn.eu/g4Ah8AO

📖 **Blood Gases**
https://www.amazon.co.uk/dp/B09755Pd1F/ref

📖 **Q & A: Anaesthetic Principles, Volume 1**
http://amzn.eu/iIbr8eK

📖 **Q & A: Anaesthetic Principles, Volume 2**
http://amzn.eu/4eKMyRe

📖 **Q & A: Anaesthetic Principles, Volume 3**
http://www.amazon.co.uk/dp/B0876F7V6S

📖 **Q & A: Anaesthetic Principles, Volumes 1-3**
https://www.amazon.co.uk/dp/B087BJ7YXW

📖 **Perioperative Topics: Test and Learn**
http://amzn.eu/gMhiDvm

📖 **Q & A: Basic Life Support**

http://amzn.eu/acoxDel

📖 **Pass Your Drug Calculation Test**

http://amzn.eu/duk6uT7

📖 **Basic Drug Calculations**

http://amzn.eu/d0SWt0c

📖 **Drug Calculation Workbook**

http://amzn.eu/d39gtl3

📖 **Drug Calculation Examples**

http://amzn.eu/76zGfkJ

📖 **Drug Calculations By Formula**

http://amzn.eu/eW9SEg3

📖 **Advanced Drug Calculation Workbook**

http://amzn.eu/7zDyFQh

📖 **Nurse Q & A: Anatomy and Physiology**

http://amzn.eu/f6nRC6G

📖 **Q & A: Respiratory System**

http://amzn.eu/7RqNNxa

Favourite Quotes

🏃 "Your best teacher is your last mistake." **Ralph Nader**.

🏃 "The mind, once enlightened, cannot again become dark." **Thomas Paine**.

🏃 "Learning is a treasure that will follow its owner everywhere." **Anonymous**.

🏃 "The beautiful thing about learning is that nobody can take it away from you." **B.B. King**.

Epilogue

The mastering of any subject, particularly drug calculations, is more a matter of perseverance and practice, rather than innate ability. For many people, who find mathematics difficult, giving up is the default behaviour, perhaps because they are emulating the attitude of others, who have also surrendered to the idea that they cannot "do" mathematics. A perceived weakness in mathematics is like a fashionable impediment, which some people seem to either flaunt, or hide, depending on their particular circumstances.

With a little determination, and a lot of commitment, especially with respect to time, anyone can gain proficiency in the basic level of mathematics needed for drug calculations.

As sages have repeated throughout the ages, "practice, practice, practice" is the mantra to follow, so that those neurological links, necessary for mastering any subject, can be formed, and which ultimately, lead to achievement.

To achieve the goal of gaining ability and confidence in calculating drug dosages for patients, it is necessary to make a personal journey of self development and, as Confucius said, "The longest journey starts with a first step"; by studying this book, you have taken that step, so don't stop until you finish the journey.

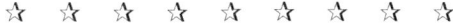

Printed in Great Britain
by Amazon

Short Stack Editions | Volume 8

Honey
by Rebekah Peppler

Short Stack Editions

Publisher: Nick Fauchald
Creative Director: Rotem Raffe
Editor: Kaitlyn Goalen
Copy Editor: Abby Tannenbaum
Wholesale Manager: Erin Fritch

ISBN 978-0-9896017-7-1

Printed in New York City
Third printing, March 2016

Table of Contents

Spreads, Slathers & Condiments

Sweets

Sips

We often describe Short Stacks as

"love letters" from an author to his or her favorite ingredient. In the case of this edition, it's more of a "love-hate" letter.

Until fairly recently, author Rebekah Peppler had nothing good to say about honey. But a transformative moment with the ingredient led her to see it in a new light and slowly emerge from her prejudice.

Although she is now firmly ensconced in the honey fan camp, make no mistake: The recipes in this book have survived the judgment of a skeptic. And in our minds, they're all the better for it.

It's clear that Rebekah's former bias acted as a powerful fuel for her work. She has dug deep to understand her change of heart, and the result is an impressively nuanced take at an overlooked ingredient. In her kitchen, honey is a category rather than a single ingredient; within that category, the applications are numerous and thoughtful.

Each recipe here is a small testimony—made by Rebekah to herself and to us—proving honey's worth. And the proof, whether in the form of popcorn spiked with *furikake*-honey butter or honey-peanut stew, more than holds up in the court of our kitchen.

Here's to happy endings,

—*The Editors*

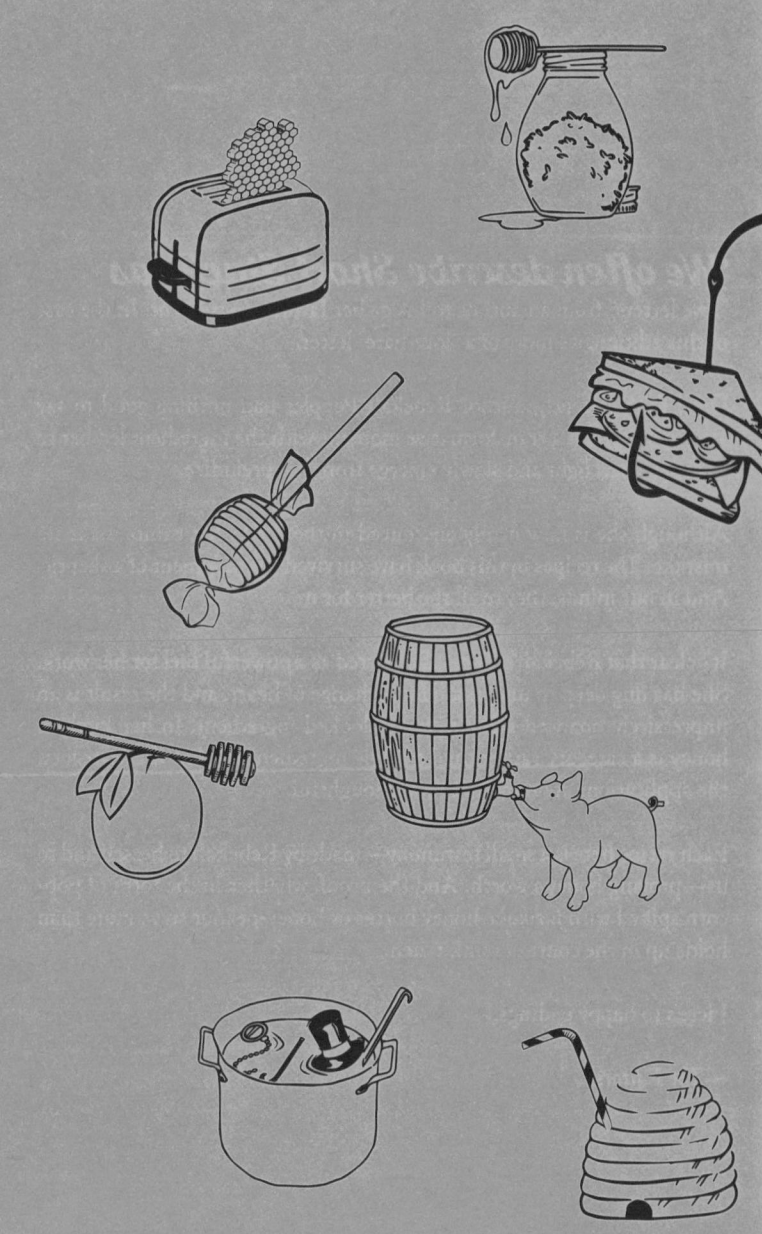

Introduction

It's an ugly truth, but let's get it out in the open: I used to hate honey.

It began in early childhood with that ubiquitous plastic honey bear. The honey's humdrum flavor, lackluster texture and pungent aftertaste fell short of the expectations a certain Pooh had set. The aversion carried through young adulthood, though in time, my feelings toward honey turned to apathy and, in deference to my line of work, I learned to tolerate and cook with honey, although without affection.

Thankfully, a moment of clarity akin to the turning point in every hero's (or in this case cookbook author's) story came to pass during a weekend I spent cooking on a working farm. The farmers were in their first year of beekeeping, and early one morning, alongside a delivery of freshly laid eggs and tender squash blossoms, sat a jar of straw-yellow honey, the first of their harvest. It was light on the tongue, delicately sweet and very fluid; it flowed off the spoon easily, as opposed to the thick, molasses texture I was accustomed to in generic store-bought honeys. Half a jar later, I sat sticky-sweet with regret: How had I let my bias against honey go unchecked for so long?

I justify my late honey conversion in this way: The one-note honey that lines the aisle of many supermarkets is not always true honey. It tends to be an unidentified mix of honeys thinned with water, blended with corn syrup and/or filtered to remove any hint of pollen. Although my honey aversion was arrogant and prolonged, I tip my hat to my younger self for realizing I was getting the short end of a very sticky stick. Markets have gotten better recently, and many now offer single-variety and wildflower honeys that can be tracked back to their source. What's more, the rise of local beekeepers and online availability of specialty honeys make first-rate honey even easier to buy.

Since that summer morning on the farm, I've opened my palate and kitchen to as many single-varietal and specialty honeys as I can get my hands on. I've discovered ways to cook with different honeys that enhance each one's inherent flavors, taking care to choose the right honey for each job. Along the way, my love for its diverse sweet and savory uses has grown exponentially. So, when I needed to choose the ingredient for this book, honey seemed the way to put my discoveries to good use—and hopefully make peace with the honey gods.

There's no lack of diversity in the world of honey, so it's an endlessly exciting ingredient for a cook. Ranging in color from pale straw to dark ebony, honey varies as widely in fragrance and flavor as it does in hue. In North America alone, there are no less than 300 unique varietals. Even the flavor profiles within each varietal are distinct from year to year and hive to hive. Similar to wine and cheese, honey is a product of its *terroir*, gleaning its character from its environment of origin.

In this edition, I chose to focus on six distinct single-varietal honeys: acacia, orange blossom, clover, tupelo, chestnut and buckwheat. This recipe collection highlights the widely ranging personalities grouped under the catchall "honey." Each recipe, both sweet and savory, includes a specific honey, chosen for its unique properties. You'll find light, buttery acacia honey mingling with Japanese *furikake* seasoning (p. 14), fruity tupelo weaving its way into baklava sticky buns (p. 35) and bittersweet chestnut transforming pork chops into sticky, bourbon-glazed knockouts (p. 27).

That said, the best part of cooking with honey is that there's an endless variety available to play with. This abbreviated set of honeys and corresponding recipes serve as just a jumping off point into the adventure of cooking with honey. I can tell you from my own exprience that once you lay aside any preconceptions and simply start tasting, a deliciously sticky world of possibilities opens up.

—*Rebekah Peppler*

Recipes

Honey Varietals

Clover

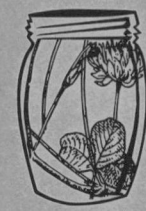

Source:	predominately white sweet clover
Color:	medium yellow to amber
Smell:	buttery, cinnamon
Flavor:	vanilla, caramel, butterscotch
Aftertaste:	mild to medium
Texture:	light to medium-bodied

Used in: Honey-Sesame Bacon (p. 12), Whole-Grain Honey Mustard (p. 29), Honeyed Pickles (p. 30), Honeycomb Candy (p. 39)

Chestnut

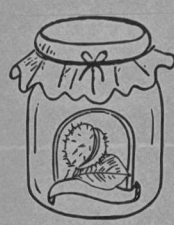

Source:	chestnut tree
Color:	dark, mahogany
Smell:	woody, animal
Flavor:	herbal, bittersweet, dark toffee
Aftertaste:	lingering, slightly bitter
Texture:	very thin, low viscosity

Used in: Pork Chops with Burnt Whiskey Honey Glaze(p. 27)

Buckwheat

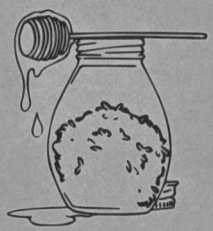

Source:	buckwheat
Color:	very dark, ebony
Smell:	malty, musty
Flavor:	assertive, molasses, dark cherries
Aftertaste:	lingering
Texture:	thick

Used in: Honey-Malt Ice Cream (p. 32), Salted Sarrasin Caramels (p. 37)

Acacia

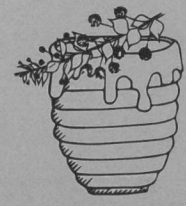

Source:	black locust tree or false acacia
Color:	light straw
Smell:	very mild
Flavor:	fresh, delicate, vanilla
Aftertaste:	mild
Texture:	light-bodied, viscous

Used in: Furikake-Honey Butter (p. 14), Furikake Popcorn (p. 15), Dutch Baby with Chamomile Honey (p. 16), Butter Lettuce with Herbed-Honey Dressing (p. 17), Riesling-Honey Jelly (p. 31)

Orange Blossom

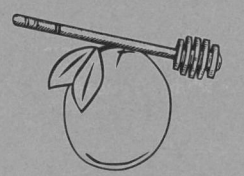

Source:	citrus/orange trees
Color:	bright yellow-orange
Smell:	floral, bright, honeysuckle
Flavor:	citrus, delicate, warm
Aftertaste:	mild, short-lasting
Texture:	medium-bodied

Used in: Roast Chicken with Lemon & Pink Pepper Honey Butter (p. 22), Bucatini with Honey-Roasted Tomatoes (p. 26), Honey-Blueberry Coffee Cake (p. 33), Orange Blossom Honey Syrup (p. 40), Bee's Knees (p. 40), Brandy Slush (p. 41) Mike's Honey-Vanilla Old-Fashioned (p. 42), Switchel (p. 43)

Tupelo

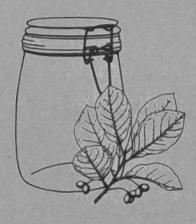

Source:	white tupelo tree
Color:	light amber
Smell:	spicy, fruit forward
Flavor:	very sweet, gently caramelized
Aftertaste:	mild, fruity
Texture:	medium body

Used in: Honey-Oat Pizza (p. 20), Friday Night Fish Sandwiches with Honey Slaw (p. 24), Baklava Sticky Buns (p. 35)

Honey-Sesame Bacon

In my house, a weekend without bacon is no weekend at all, but even the tastiest things are not exempt from becoming monotonous. Enter honey-sesame bacon: Imbued with the same flavors as takeout Chinese sesame chicken, it injects just the right amount of savory-sweet variation into the bacon circuit. Eat it as is or layer it with ripe tomato slices and lettuce between toasted white bread for a superior BLT.

1 pound thick-cut bacon

½ cup clover honey

Pinch cayenne pepper

1 tablespoon white sesame seeds, divided

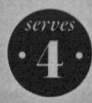

serves
·4·

Preheat the oven to 400°. Line a rimmed baking sheet with nonstick aluminum foil and arrange the bacon slices in a single layer. Bake until the fat is rendered and the bacon begins to crisp, about 15 minutes.

Meanwhile, in a small saucepan over medium heat, heat the honey, cayenne and half of the sesame seeds until warmed through. Remove the baking sheet from the oven, carefully drain off some of the bacon fat and brush the honey mixture over the bacon slices. Return the bacon to the oven and bake until the glaze is bubbling and the bacon is crisp, 5 to 7 minutes. Sprinkle the remaining sesame seeds over the bacon and transfer to a paper-towel-lined plate, lacquered side up. Serve warm.

Honeycomb Toasts

Warm buttered bread, though straightforward, is one of my favorite treats. This recipe elevates the simple combination to deity status by adding thick chucks of comb honey on top. Comb honey is honey that's still encased in its original beeswax cells, and it's perfectly edible. The comb's chewy, waxy texture contrasts nicely with the smooth honey and softens slightly on the warm bread. And don't skimp on the butter: A thick layer acts as an anchor for the honeycomb and balances out the unfettered sweetness.

1 small honeycomb (about 8 ounces), cut into pieces (available at specialty stores and farmers' markets)

Four 1-inch-thick slices country bread

1 stick (8 tablespoons) salted European butter, at room temperature

Flaky sea salt (optional)

Ground cardamom (optional)

makes 4 toasts

Toast the bread in a toaster or under the broiler. Slather each slice evenly with a thick layer of butter. Top each slice with a piece of honeycomb and drizzle with any excess honey. Sprinkle with sea salt and cardamom, if using. Serve warm.

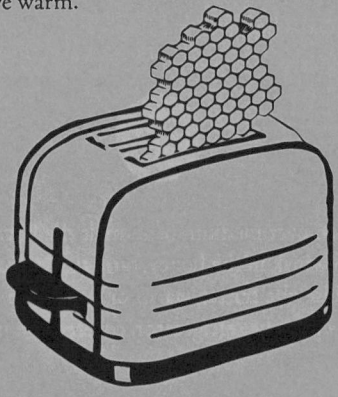

Furikake-Honey Butter

A few days after a recent trip to Paris, I sat in my tiny Brooklyn apartment while a chilly autumn rain pounded against the window. Coming down from a travel high is never pleasant, but this time it seemed exceptionally acute, if only for all the over-the-top bread, cheese and butter I could no longer get my hands on. I rummaged through the cabinets, hungry and pining for something to fill the void, when I came across a jar of *furikake*. The Japanese seasoning, made with toasted seaweed and sesame seeds, called to mind one French butter in particular: Jean-Yves Bordier's celebrated *beurre aux algues* (seaweed butter). Adding a quick whisk of *furikake* into melted honey butter seamlessly infused the fat with a sweet, saline flavor. It's delicious on a crisp French baguette; popcorn is also an ideal bedfellow (see p.15). The versatile infused butter is equally at home brushed over seared scallops, tossed with baby potatoes or stirred into homemade snack mix.

1 stick (8 tablespoons) unsalted butter

1 tablespoon acacia honey

1 tablespoon *furikake* seasoning (available at Asian markets or online)

1 tablespoon flaky sea salt

makes 2/3 *cup*

In a small saucepan over medium heat, melt the butter. Remove the pan from the heat and whisk in the honey, *furikake* and salt, stirring until the honey dissolves. Use the butter warm or pour into ramekins and chill. The butter will keep in the refrigerator, covered, for up to 1 month.

Furikake Popcorn

2 tablespoons vegetable oil
⅔ cup popcorn kernels
⅔ cup *furikake* butter (p.14)

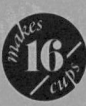

In a large saucepan or Dutch oven, heat the oil over medium-high heat until it shimmers. Add the popcorn kernels, shake to coat in oil and cover. Cook, shaking the pot occasionally, until all the kernels have popped, 5 to 7 minutes. Transfer the popcorn to a large bowl; discard any unpopped kernels. Drizzle the *furikake* butter over the popcorn, tossing gently to coat; serve warm.

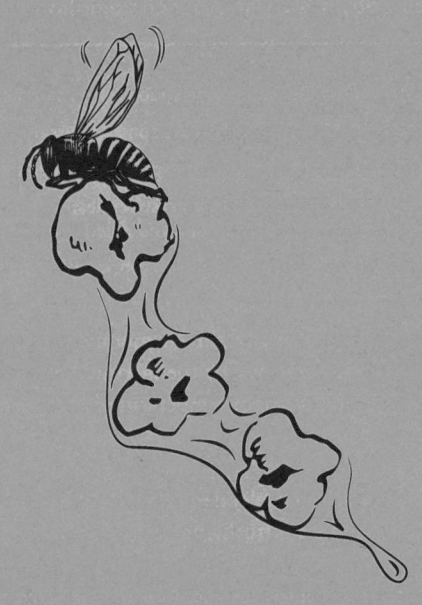

Dutch Baby
with Chamomile Honey

Dutch baby, Dutch puff, *pannenkoek*, Bismarck: Whatever you call it, this brunch powerhouse pancake is one of the easiest week-end-worthy breakfasts this side of room service. Its light texture and buttery flavor leave acacia's herbal flavors room to shine, especially if you start the chamomile infusion earlier in the week. That said, if you come across a jar of raspberry honey, snap it up and infuse that instead: Paired with the fresh raspberries embed-ded in the Dutch baby, it's a knockout combination.

1 tablespoon dried chamomile, coarsely chopped

½ cup acacia honey

3 large eggs

½ cup all-purpose flour

½ cup whole milk

¾ teaspoon pure vanilla extract

¼ teaspoon kosher salt

2 tablespoons unsalted butter

1 cup raspberries, rinsed and dried

½ lemon (optional)

serves **4**

Make the chamomile honey: Place the chamomile in the bottom of a clean glass jar and add the honey. Stir the mixture with a clean spoon. Cover tightly and set aside at room temperature for at least 4 days and up to 1 month.

Preheat the oven to 425°. In a blender, combine the eggs, flour, milk, vanilla and salt and blend until frothy, about 1 minute.

Set a 10-inch cast-iron skillet over medium heat and add the butter. Heat, tilting the pan to coat it evenly, until the butter is melted and bubbling. Add the raspberries to the skillet and pour the batter on top; immediately transfer the skillet to the oven. Bake until puffed and golden around the edges, 18 to 22 minutes.

Remove the Dutch baby from the oven and transfer it to a large plate. Drizzle with chamomile honey and the freshly squeezed juice of the lemon half, if desired. Cut into wedges and serve immediately.

Butter Lettuce with Herbed-Honey Dressing

Tender butter lettuce doesn't benefit from thick, goopy dressing. Mild acacia honey gives this herby vinaigrette body but not heft: It clings to the leaves lightly without weighing them down.

3 teaspoons acacia honey

½ lemon, zested and juiced (about 2 tablespoons juice)

½ teaspoon Dijon mustard

2 tablespoons flat-leaf parsley leaves, plus 1 teaspoon finely chopped

2 tablespoons torn basil leaves, plus 1 teaspoon finely chopped basil

¼ cup extra-virgin olive oil

Kosher salt and freshly ground black pepper

1 large head butter lettuce, cored, leaves torn into bite-size pieces

3 radishes, thinly sliced

serves · 4 ·

In a small bowl, whisk together the honey, lemon juice and zest, mustard, chopped parsley and chopped basil until combined. Gradually add the olive oil, whisking constantly, until a creamy, emulsified dressing forms. Season with salt and pepper.

Place the butter lettuce, radishes, parsley leaves and torn basil leaves in a large bowl. Drizzle with the dressing and toss gently to coat. Season with salt and pepper and serve.

Honey-Roasted Peanut Stew

Be warned: I've never actually tasted this stew, though I've made it enough times to know the recipe by heart. A few years ago, I developed a sudden, intense peanut allergy and am still grieving the abrupt departure of my breakfast stalwart: peanut butter toast drizzled with honey. But, knowing the matchless union between peanut butter and honey, I can't deprive the rest of you good, non-ground-nut-sensitive folks the pleasure. Enter this honey-roasted peanut stew. It's ridiculously simple to prepare, makes your kitchen smell *amazing* and, as my taste-tester friends can attest (with a tad too much gusto for my or my allergist's liking), the resulting potage is sweet, thick and teeming with caramelized, peanut-y flavor. The stew is ideal for ladling over cooked rice; serve with lime wedges to cut through the its gentle sweetness.

1 cup honey-roasted peanuts

1 tablespoon canola or peanut oil

1 medium yellow onion, finely chopped

3 garlic cloves, finely chopped

One 1-inch piece fresh ginger, peeled and finely chopped

1 teaspoon ground cumin

½ teaspoon ground coriander

¾ teaspoon kosher salt, plus more to taste

¼ teaspoon cayenne pepper

6 cups low-sodium vegetable broth

1 medium sweet potato, diced

1 small bunch cilantro, stems and leaves divided, stems tied with twine

¼ cup tomato paste

1 bunch kale, ribs removed and leaves sliced crosswise into 1-inch strips

4 cups cooked brown rice

1 lime, cut into wedges

serves
·4·

Add the peanuts to a food processor and pulse until coarsely chopped. Transfer ¼ cup of chopped peanuts to a small bowl and set aside; continue blending the remaining peanuts until a smooth paste forms, about 4 minutes. Set aside.

In a large Dutch oven over medium heat, heat the oil until shimmering. Add the onion, garlic and ginger and cook, stirring, until they have softened, 7 to 10 minutes. Add the cumin, coriander, salt and cayenne pepper and stir to combine. Add the vegetable broth and bring to a simmer. Add the sweet potato and cilantro stems. Simmer, stirring occasionally, until the sweet potato cubes are just tender, 15 to 20 minutes.

In a medium mixing bowl, whisk together the peanut butter and tomato paste. Ladle 2 cups of the hot broth into the peanut butter mixture and whisk until smooth. Transfer the mixture to the Dutch oven and stir to combine. Simmer for 10 minutes, then remove the cilantro and stir in the kale. Continue simmering until the kale is tender and wilted, 8 to 10 minutes. Season to taste with salt. Divide the rice among bowls and top with stew. Garnish with the cilantro leaves and reserved chopped peanuts. Serve with lime wedges.

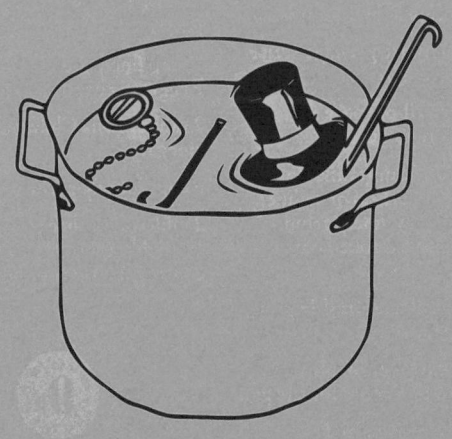

Honey-Oat Pizza with Taleggio, Arugula and Bee Pollen

Despite my childhood dislike for all things honey, Honey Nut Cheerios featured heavily and happily in the breakfasts of my youth. This pizza dough honors the best of those sweet, oat-y rounds (without all the added sugar). Topped with pungent Talegio cheese, lightly dressed arugula and a sprinkle of floral bee pollen, this pizza has become my new favorite meal—morning, noon or night. For a truly dawn-friendly feast, crack an egg or two on top during the last 5 minutes of baking.

If you have pollen allergies, use caution when trying bee pollen for the first time. Look for pollen from a local beekeeper and begin by tasting it in very small amounts (¼ teaspoon at a time) before working up to a larger amount. If your allergies are severe, consult a physician before ingesting.

1 cup lukewarm water, divided

¼ cup tupelo honey, divided

One ¼-ounce package active dry yeast

2¾ cups all-purpose flour, plus more to dust

1 cup oat flour (available at gourmet markets or online; alternatively, finely grind old-fashioned rolled oats in a food processor)

Kosher salt and freshly ground black pepper

¾ cup extra-virgin olive oil, divided, plus more for the pan

1 garlic clove, halved

1 pound Taleggio cheese, rind removed, cheese cut into small pieces

½ cup finely grated Parmigiano-Reggiano cheese

2 tablespoons Champagne vinegar

8 cups loosely packed arugula

2 tablespoons bee pollen (available at health stores, gourmet markets or online)

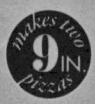

In a large bowl, combine ½ cup of the lukewarm water and 1 tablespoon of the honey; whisk to dissolve the honey. Sprinkle the yeast over the surface and set aside until the mixture is foaming and bubbling, about 5 minutes.

In a medium bowl, whisk together the all-purpose flour, oat flour and 1 teaspoon of salt. Add the flour mixture to the yeast along with the remaining ½ cup of water and ¼ cup plus 2 tablespoons of olive oil and stir to combine. Turn the dough out onto a lightly floured work surface and knead until the dough is smooth and elastic, 5 to 8 minutes. Transfer the dough to a lightly oiled bowl and cover with plastic wrap. Set aside in a warm spot until the dough has doubled in size, about 1 hour.

Punch the dough down, return to the bowl, cover with plastic wrap and set aside to rise a second time, until the dough has again doubled in size, about 1 hour. Divide the dough into 2 equal discs, place them on a work surface and cover each loosely with plastic wrap. Let the dough rest for 30 minutes, then lightly flour the work surface and use the heels of your hands to gently stretch each disc into a 9-inch round. Transfer each to a lightly oiled baking sheet.

Preheat the oven to 400°. Lightly brush each pizza crust with 1 table-spoon of the olive oil. Bake until the crusts are firm and lightly golden, about 10 minutes. Remove the crusts from the oven and rub each with the cut sides of the garlic clove. Scatter the Taleggio evenly over both pizzas and sprinkle each with ¼ cup of Parmigiano-Reggiano. Return to the oven and bake until the crusts are golden brown and the cheese is bubbly, 5 to 7 minutes.

In a large bowl, whisk together ¼ cup of the olive oil and the Champagne vinegar; season with salt and pepper to taste. Add the arugula and toss to coat. Sprinkle each pizza with 1 tablespoon of bee pollen and drizzle with the remaining honey. Mound the dressed arugula in the center of each pizza and serve immediately.

Roast Chicken with Lemon & Pink Pepper Honey Butter

Sweet as honey is, it slides into a savory role easily. The key lies in pairing it with other ingredients that boost its flavor profile while tempering its sweetness. Orange blossom honey, used here, is prized for its fruity, citrus notes; when it's paired with spicy, citric pink peppercorns and Meyer lemon, it makes a superlative rub for roast chicken. The honey butter is tucked under the chicken's skin before roasting and brushed on top while it cooks, creating a one-two punch of tender, flavorful meat and peppery, lacquered skin. Make extra pink peppercorn honey butter and brush it over grilled corn, spread it on waffles or spoon it over roasted sweet potatoes.

5 tablespoons unsalted butter, at room temperature

2 tablespoons orange blossom honey

2 teaspoons freshly ground pink peppercorns (from 1 tablespoon whole peppercorns)

1 small Meyer lemon, finely zested, then thinly sliced

Kosher salt

One 4-pound chicken

1 garlic clove, peeled and smashed

serves
·4·

Preheat the oven to 375°. In a medium bowl, combine the butter, honey, pink peppercorns and Meyer lemon zest. Season lightly with salt and mix to combine. Use your fingers to carefully loosen the skin from the chicken breast and spread half of the butter under the skin. Season the entire chicken, including the cavity, with salt.

Fill the chicken cavity with the lemon slices and garlic and tie the legs loosely with twine. Place the chicken, breast side up, on a rack fitted inside a small roasting pan; roast for 30 minutes. Pour ¼ cup of water into the roasting pan and, using a pastry brush, brush the chicken with some of the remaining butter mixture; return to the oven. Continue roasting, brushing the chicken with the butter every 10 minutes, until an instant-read thermometer inserted into the thickest part of a thigh reaches 165°, 35 to 40 minutes more. Carefully remove the chicken from the oven, transfer to a cutting board and let rest for 10 to 15 minutes before carving and serving.

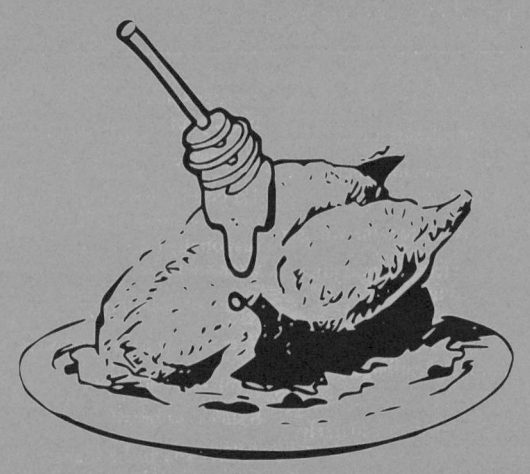

Friday Night Fish Sandwiches with Honey Slaw

Growing up in Wisconsin, I spent many Friday nights tucked into a wood-paneled booth downing Shirley Temples and joining in a Midwestern tradition: the Friday Night Fish Fry. This recipe takes the elements of that event—crispy, beer-battered fillets of fresh-water fish, creamy coleslaw and slices of rye bread—and piles them into one satisfying sandwich. Tupelo honey, which has a higher-than-average fructose content that lends it an incredibly smooth texture and heightened sweetness, imbues the slaw with a light butterscotch-y flavor. Serve alongside a Shirley Temple—strike that, an old-fashioned (made with brandy, of course)—and toast to a vital Midwest tradition.

½ cup mayonnaise

2 teaspoons Dijon mustard

2 teaspoons tupelo honey, plus more to finish

2 teaspoons white wine vinegar

2 teaspoons fresh lemon juice, plus more to finish

¼ teaspoon hot sauce

½ medium red cabbage, thinly sliced

2 carrots, peeled and coarsely grated

Kosher salt and freshly ground black pepper

Vegetable oil, for frying

1½ pounds boneless, skinless perch or cod fillets, sliced diagonally into 1½-inch-wide strips

1 cup Wondra flour

½ teaspoon baking powder

1 cup lager-style beer

8 slices rye bread

4 slices sharp cheddar cheese, preferably Wisconsin cheddar

makes
4

In a large bowl, whisk together the mayonnaise, mustard, honey, vinegar, lemon juice and hot sauce. Add the cabbage and carrots and toss to coat. Season with salt and pepper. Cover the coleslaw with plastic wrap and refrigerate while you make the fish.

Fill a large saucepan halfway with oil and heat over medium-high heat until it reaches 350° on a digital thermometer. Line a baking sheet or large plate with paper towels and set aside.

While the oil is heating, place the flour and baking powder in a medium shallow bowl; whisk together until well combined. Season generously with salt and pepper. Slowly pour in the beer, whisking until a smooth batter forms.

Season the fish with salt. Working in batches, dip each piece into the batter and coat completely. Shake off any excess batter and place the fish in the hot oil. Fry the fish, using a slotted spoon to turn the fillets occasionally, until they are golden brown and crisp, 7 to 8 minutes. Using a slotted spoon, transfer the fish to the paper-towel-lined plate and season with salt. Repeat with the remaining fish and batter.

Lightly toast the bread and top four with the cheddar slices. Divide the fish among the slices of cheese-covered toast, then drizzle them with honey and top with coleslaw. Cover with the remaining toast and serve warm.

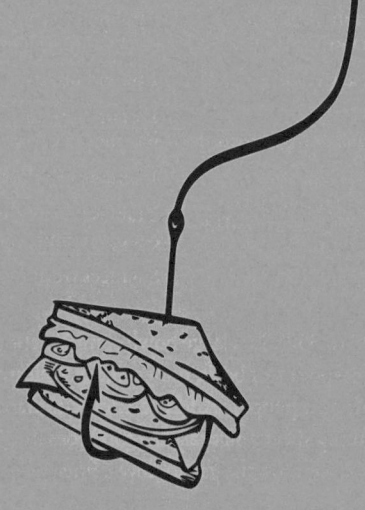

Bucatini with Honey-Roasted Tomatoes

A last-minute addition to the book, this recipe quickly ascended to the top of my weeknight repertoire. As it turns out, roasting cherry tomatoes in orange blossom honey (and plenty of herbs) boosts their flavor during the off-season and further amps up their sweetness in season, all the while transforming them into a jammy mess of awesomeness. Tossing the tomatoes with bucatini (a pasta slightly fatter than spaghetti, with a hollow center) produces a dish that sings of summer all year round. For another meal, scrap the pasta and serve the roasted tomatoes alongside salmon fillets or pile atop crusty bread slathered with ricotta. When I retested the recipe, I also found the ruptured tomatoes make a brilliant addition to a slab of honey-oat pizza (p. 20).

3 garlic cloves, peeled and smashed

¼ cup coarsely chopped flat-leaf parsley, divided

¼ cup coarsely chopped basil, divided

2 tablespoons orange blossom honey

¼ cup plus 2 tablespoons extra-virgin olive oil, divided

Kosher salt and freshly ground black pepper

2 pounds cherry tomatoes, halved

1 pound bucatini

1½ cups grated Parmigiano-Reggiano

1 lemon, zested and juiced

2 tablespoons coarsely chopped mint

8 ounces fresh ricotta

serves **4**

Preheat the oven to 350°. In a large bowl, combine the garlic, 2 tablespoons of parsley, 2 tablespoons of basil, honey and 2 tablespoons of the olive oil. Season with salt and pepper. Add the cherry tomatoes and toss to coat. Transfer to a baking sheet and roast the tomatoes until they begin to burst, 18 to 22 minutes. Remove the garlic cloves, finely chop them and set aside.

Cook the pasta in a large pot of boiling, salted water until al dente. Drain, reserving 1 cup of the cooking liquid; transfer the pasta to a large bowl. Add ½ cup of the reserved cooking liquid, the remaining ¼ cup of olive oil, the Parmigiano-Reggiano, lemon juice and zest, the remaining parsley and basil and the mint and toss to coat. Add the tomatoes, chopped garlic and any juices to the bowl and toss just to combine. In another bowl, season the ricotta with salt and pepper.

Divide the pasta among bowls, dollop with some of the ricotta, season with pepper and serve.

Pork Chops with Burnt Whiskey Honey Glaze

As with sugar, the process of caramelizing honey deepens its flavors and tempers its sweetness. I like to use the technique with chestnut honey in particular; doing so brings out its tobacco-y and bittersweet flavors, leading it into the realm of the savory. Infusing the honey with whiskey, orange peel and peppercorns further heightens those flavors into a smoky, sticky glaze that's ideal for coating thick, oven-roasted pork chops. Moreover, it provides a good excuse for serving a finger or two of whiskey with dinner.

½ cup chestnut honey

¼ cup bourbon or rye whiskey

1 orange peel, cut into large pieces, pith removed

¼ teaspoon whole black peppercorns

Pinch cayenne pepper

Four 1- to 1¼-inch-thick pork rib chops

Kosher salt and freshly ground black pepper

2 tablespoons vegetable oil

serves 4

In a medium saucepan over medium heat, warm the honey, stirring occasionally, until it is fragrant and has darkened slightly in color, about 5 minutes. Stir in the whiskey, orange peel, peppercorns and cayenne pepper and remove the pan from the heat; set aside to cool. Once the honey mixture has cooled, strain it through a fine-mesh sieve into a bowl.

Pat the pork chops dry with a paper towel and season generously with salt and pepper. Place on a plate and set aside for 15 minutes.

Meanwhile, preheat the oven to 350°. Set a large cast-iron skillet or two medium cast-iron skillets over high heat. Add the oil and heat until shimmering. Add the pork chops and sear on one side, without moving, until deep golden brown, about 4 minutes. Flip the chops and sear the second side until golden brown, 3 to 4 minutes. Brush the pork chops with some of the bourbon-honey glaze and transfer the skillet to the oven. Roast, brushing the pork chops occasionally with additional glaze, until an instant-read thermometer inserted into the meat registers 145°, 18 to 22 minutes. Transfer the pork chops to a serving platter, brush with any remaining glaze and let rest, uncovered, for 15 minutes before serving.

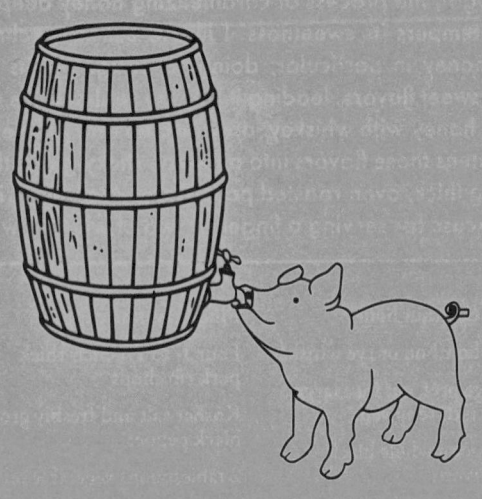

Whole-Grain
Honey Mustard

A while back, as I was assembling a rather ordinary turkey sand-wich, I pulled out my go-to jar of honey mustard. With my knife hovering above the jar, I realized that I wanted its sweetness but also the characteristic pop of a whole-grain mustard. I Mac-Gyvered a mix of the two, vowing to create the condiment I truly craved from scratch at a later date. Although you'll have to exer-cise a bit of patience, give the mustard time to rest before serving (one to two weeks is best). The result: an intensely flavored and textured spread that aspires to rise a notch above and beyond that humble lunchtime condiment. Whisked into a hyper-vinegary potato salad, brushed over salmon fillets or served alongside charcuterie, this mustard's possibilities are endless.

¼ cup yellow mustard seeds

¼ cup brown mustard seeds

½ cup Champagne vinegar

¼ cup dry white wine

½ teaspoon kosher salt

¼ cup clover honey

makes 1¼ cups

In a medium bowl, combine the yellow and brown mustard seeds, vine-gar, wine and kosher salt. Cover the bowl with plastic wrap and let it sit at room temperature overnight. Transfer 2 tablespoons of the mustard seed mixture into a small bowl and set aside. Transfer the rest to a food processor along with the honey. Process the mustard until it's creamy. Use a spatula to stir in the reserved seeds. Transfer the mustard to a covered container and refrigerate for at least 1 week. Stored in the refrig-erator, the mustard will keep for up to 3 months.

Honeyed Pickles

Skirting the line between classic dills and bread-and-butters, these spears sweeten over time. Clover honey, America's most common single-varietal honey, is a team player and won't overpower the brine. Since nobody likes a limp pickle, use these tricks to keep your pickles crisp.

One:
Use the freshest cucumbers you can find; they're as crisp and firm as they ever will be.

Two:
Trim the ends off your cucumbers before packing them into the jars. The blossom end contains an enzyme that can lead to softening.

Three:
Don't boil the jars in water to seal the lids. The heat that facilitates canning also cooks the pickles slightly. Refrigerator pickles aren't shelf stable, but they do keep for a while in the fridge. Simply make another batch when you're running low.

---

1 pound Kirby cucumbers (about 3 medium), quartered lengthwise

10 dill sprigs

2 garlic cloves, peeled and smashed

¾ cup apple cider vinegar

¾ cup water

¼ cup clover honey

1½ tablespoons kosher salt

2 teaspoons whole yellow mustard seeds

½ teaspoon black peppercorns

¼ teaspoon red pepper flakes

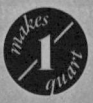

Fill a large-mouthed quart jar with the cucumbers, dill and garlic.

In a saucepan over medium heat, combine the vinegar, water, honey, salt, mustard seeds, peppercorns and red pepper flakes. Bring the mixture to a simmer, stirring to dissolve the honey. Pour the mixture over the cucumbers and refrigerate, uncovered, for 24 hours. Cover and refrigerate the pickles for an additional 24 hours before serving. The pickles will keep, in the refrigerator, for up to two weeks.

Riesling-Honey Jelly

Dry Riesling and acacia honey have surprisingly parallel flavor profiles. Sweet, buttery and light, they play off each other in the most pleasant of ways. Fashioned into a jelly and cut with a splash of lemon juice, the combination will instantly refine a cheese plate. I've also been known to spread the stuff over crusty, buttered toast or drop a spoonful into a glass of bubbly.

2 cups dry Riesling

1 lemon, juiced
(about 2 tablespoons)

¼ cup acacia honey

One 1¾-ounce package
powdered fruit pectin

In a medium saucepan over medium-high heat, bring the wine to a simmer. Add the lemon juice and honey and stir to combine. Add the pectin and boil, whisking constantly, for 2 minutes. Remove the pan from the heat and use a spoon to skim off any foam that rises to the surface. Pour the mixture into two 8-ounce sterilized glass jars, cover and refrigerate until the jelly is set, at least 12 hours. Refrigerate for up to 3 weeks.

Honey-Malt Ice Cream

In high school, my best friend and I would meet regularly for an after-school snack of extra-thick malted milk shakes and fried cheese curds. Those days (and that metabolism) are long gone, but our love of malt remains strong. For a decidedly more adult version, I add thick, musty buckwheat honey to double down on the malty, chocolaty flavor. Serve the ice cream as is, drizzle scoops with additional buckwheat honey and top with toasted pecans, or add to a blender with a splash of whole milk for a milkshake that will haunt your dreams.

⅓ cup buckwheat honey

1 cup whole milk

2 cups heavy cream

⅓ cup malted milk powder

¼ teaspoon kosher salt

5 large egg yolks

3 tablespoons granulated sugar

makes 1 quart

In a large saucepan over medium-high heat, warm the honey until it's smooth and heated through, about 1 minute. Gradually pour in the milk and cream, whisking constantly until combined. Whisk in the malted milk powder and salt and cook until barely simmering.

In a medium bowl, whisk together the egg yolks and sugar until the yolks turn a pale yellow color. Gradually pour half of the honey-cream mixture into the eggs, whisking constantly, until the egg mixture is warmed through. Add the egg-cream mixture to the pan and set over medium-low heat. Cook, stirring constantly with a wooden spoon, until the mixture is thick and coats the back of the spoon, 8 to 10 minutes. Strain the custard through a fine-mesh sieve into a large, clean bowl. Place a sheet of plastic wrap directly on the surface of the custard and refrigerate until chilled, at least 6 hours and up to overnight.

Freeze in an ice-cream machine according to manufacturer's instructions. Store in an airtight plastic container in the freezer for up to two weeks.

Honey-Blueberry Coffee Cake

Coffee cake is one of my favorite morning baking projects, mainly because it justifies eating large quantities of dessert for breakfast. This cake hits all the high points: a tender, moist crumb, pops of sweet berries and plenty of buttery, crisp streusel. Substitute blueberry honey for the aromatic orange blossom variety if you come across it.

For the streusel:

¾ cup all-purpose flour

⅓ cup granulated sugar

1 teaspoon instant espresso powder

¼ teaspoon kosher salt

5 tablespoons unsalted butter, chilled and cubed

½ cup chopped walnuts

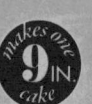

For the cake:

2 cups all-purpose flour, plus more for the pan

1 teaspoon baking powder

1 teaspoon ground cardamom

½ teaspoon kosher salt

2 sticks (one cup) unsalted butter, melted, plus more for the pan

½ cup orange blossom honey

1½ cups granulated sugar

1 cup sour cream

2 large eggs, at room temperature

Finely grated zest of 1 orange

1½ teaspoons pure vanilla extract

1 cup fresh blueberries, rinsed and dried

Preheat the oven to 350°. Butter and flour a 9-inch springform pan with a removable bottom and tap out the excess flour.

Make the streusel: In a medium bowl, mix together the flour, sugar, espresso powder and salt. Add the butter and, using your fingers, mix until the streusel clumps together in large crumbs. Mix in the walnuts and set aside.

Make the cake: In a medium bowl, whisk together the flour, baking powder, cardamom and salt and set aside.

In a large bowl, combine the butter, honey, sugar, sour cream, eggs, orange zest and vanilla and whisk until well combined. Add the flour mixture and mix just until combined, taking care not to overmix. Spread half of the batter in the prepared pan and sprinkle evenly with the blueberries. Top with the remaining batter, then sprinkle with the streusel. Bake, rotating the pan once, until the cake is golden brown, springs back when gently pressed and a toothpick inserted in the center comes out clean, about 1 hour and 30 minutes. Let the cake cool for 1 hour in the pan, then remove the sides of the springform pan and let it cool completely before cutting into wedges and serving.

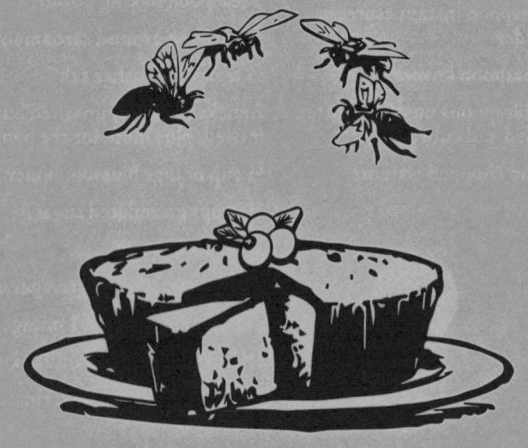

Baklava Sticky Buns

This is the first recipe I wrote for this book. It's also the very last recipe I finished, and for good reason: The road to these sticky-sweet, pistachio-laced buns is long, involved and very much worth the trouble. To develop the final recipe printed here, I started slowly, tweaking each batch in turn to balance the levels of sweet, spice, crunch and stickiness until the buns mirrored the layered flavors and textures of traditional baklava. The result is exactly what I imagined when I wrote the recipe title: rich, deeply sweet and outrageously sticky.

For the dough:

2½ cups all-purpose flour

½ cup finely ground pistachios

¼ cup granulated sugar

½ teaspoon kosher salt

⅓ cup warm whole milk

⅓ cup warm water

1 tablespoon tupelo honey

One ¼-ounce package active dry yeast

1 large egg, at room temperature

1 large egg yolk, at room temperature

10 tablespoons (1 stick plus 2 tablespoons) unsalted butter, cut into small pieces, at room temperature, plus more for the pan

For the filling:

1 cup light brown sugar

1½ teaspoons ground cinnamon

½ teaspoon ground cardamom

Finely grated zest of 1 lemon

2 tablespoons unsalted butter, melted, plus more for the pan

2 tablespoons tupelo honey

½ cup coarsely chopped pistachios

For the glaze:

⅔ cup tupelo honey

6 tablespoons (¾ stick) unsalted butter, at room temperature

2 tablespoons light brown sugar

½ cup coarsely chopped pistachios

1 teaspoon flaky sea salt

makes 8 buns

Make the dough: In a bowl, whisk together the flour, ground pistachios, sugar and salt; set aside. Place the milk, water and honey in the bowl of a stand mixer and whisk at low speed until the honey dissolves. Sprinkle the yeast over the mixture and set aside until the yeast is foamy, about 5 minutes. Add the egg and yolk, whisking until they've been incorporated into the mixture. Fit the mixer with the dough hook and, with the mixer running at medium-low speed, add the flour mixture and mix until combined. Increase the speed to medium, add the butter one or two pieces at a time, mixing until each addition is completely incorporated before adding more. The dough should be very soft and smooth. Increase the speed to medium high and continue to beat the dough until it pulls away from the sides of the bowl, 6 to 8 minutes. Transfer the dough to a large, lightly greased bowl. Cover with plastic wrap and set aside in a warm place until the dough doubles in size, 1 to 1½ hours. (At this point, the dough can be punched down and refrigerated up to overnight.)

Make the filling: In a small bowl, whisk together the brown sugar, cinnamon, cardamom and lemon zest. Set aside.

Generously butter a 9-by-13-inch pan. Dust a work surface generously with flour. Punch down the dough and transfer it to the prepared surface; knead until the dough is no longer sticky, about 1 minute, dusting with additional flour as needed. Use a floured rolling pin to roll the dough into a 10-by-20-inch rectangle that's about ¼-inch thick. Brush the dough with 2 tablespoons of melted butter and sprinkle with the brown sugar mixture, leaving a 1-inch border on the long edge closest to you. Drizzle the dough with 2 tablespoons of honey and sprinkle the ½ cup of the chopped pistachios over the dough. Starting with the edge closest to you, roll the dough lengthwise into a tight log; stop when the seam side faces down. Use a knife to cut the log into 8 equal pieces and transfer them to the prepared pan, laying them flat so that the spiral faces up. Cover the pan with plastic wrap and set aside in a warm place until the buns have doubled in size, 1 to 1½ hours.

Make the glaze: In a small saucepan over medium heat, whisk together the honey, butter and sugar and heat until the butter has melted and the sugar has dissolved, 3 to 5 minutes. Set aside.

Preheat the oven to 350°. Place the rested buns in the oven and bake until they're golden and puffed, 30 to 35 minutes. Remove the pan from the oven and brush the buns with half of the honey glaze. Return to the oven and bake until the glaze is glossy and bubbling, about 5 minutes longer. Brush with the remaining glaze, sprinkle with the ½ cup of chopped pistachios and the sea salt and let cool slightly. Serve warm or at room temperature.

Salted Sarrasin Caramels

I ate my first *sarrasin* (buckwheat) caramel on a tiny side street in Paris and was immediately smitten with the dark, buttery confection. Here, I add buckwheat honey to traditional butter caramels to create a dense, earthy sweet that borders on the happy cusp of bitter. A final shower of sea salt helps bolster the richness of the caramel and adds a subtle-yet-vital crunch. Here's something to keep in mind for making caramels: Once the honey and sugar melt, stir the caramel only as much as necessary to keep the mixture smooth. Overstirring causes the sugars to crystallize and yields a less-than-optimal caramel.

¾ cup heavy cream

1 vanilla bean, split and scraped (pod reserved for another use)

1 teaspoon flaky sea salt, plus more to finish

⅓ cup buckwheat honey

1½ cups granulated sugar

5 tablespoons unsalted butter, cubed, at room temperature

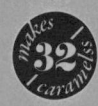

Line an 8-inch-square baking pan with parchment paper, leaving an overhang on two opposite sides; coat with nonstick spray.

In a medium saucepan over medium-high heat, combine the cream, vanilla bean seeds and salt and bring just to a boil. Remove the pan from the heat, cover and keep warm while you make the syrup.

In a large saucepan over medium heat, combine the honey and sugar. Heat, stirring occasionally, until the sugar dissolves, about 3 minutes. Continue to cook, without stirring, until the mixture reaches 300° on a candy thermometer, 8 to 10 minutes.

Gradually add the cubed butter to the caramel, whisking to combine. Once all the butter has been incorporated, slowly whisk in the cream mixture and stir just until smooth. Continue to cook, without stirring, until the caramel reaches 265° on a candy thermometer, 15 to 20 minutes. Immediately pour the caramel into the prepared pan. Cool for 15 minutes, then sprinkle with additional salt. Let cool at room temperature for at least 6 hours or up to overnight.

Once the candy has cooled, remove the caramel from the pan using the parchment overhang, then cut into 1-inch-by-2-inch rectangles. Wrap each caramel in wax paper and store in an airtight container for up to 1 month.

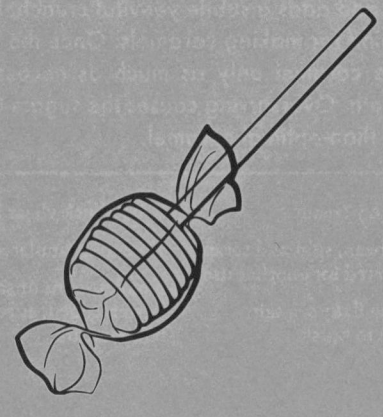

Honeycomb Candy

Honeycomb candy entered my life when I was studying abroad in England, where I basically lived on Crunchie bars and pints of ale. Back home, I craved the golden, airy confection and took to the kitchen to recreate it. Also called sea foam, sponge candy or Hokey Pokey, the honeycomb candy can be served plain or dipped in melted dark chocolate for the ultimate Crunchie experience. I time making batches so I can send candy home with friends and spare myself the indignity of eating the entire pan in one sitting. Don't say you haven't been warned.

1 tablespoon baking soda	1½ cups granulated sugar
1 teaspoon finely grated ginger	¼ cup clover honey
¼ teaspoon ground ginger	¼ teaspoon flaky sea salt

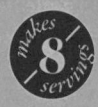

Line a rimmed baking sheet with parchment paper and spray with non-stick spray. Alternatively, line the baking sheet with a nonstick baking mat. In a small bowl, whisk together the baking soda, grated ginger and ground ginger; set aside.

In a large heavy saucepan over medium-high heat, combine the sugar, honey and ¼ cup of water. Heat, stirring, until the sugar dissolves, about 5 minutes. Continue cooking, without stirring, until the caramel is dark amber in color and reaches 300° on a candy thermometer, 8 to 10 minutes. Immediately remove the pan from the heat and carefully whisk in the baking-soda-ginger mixture (the mixture will bubble up vigorously). Working quickly, pour the mixture onto the prepared baking sheet. (Do not spread the mixture into an even layer, as doing so will cause air bubbles to form. The caramel will settle itself out as it cools). Sprinkle with sea salt and set aside to cool completely, about 20 minutes. Break the candy into large pieces. Store in an airtight container for up to 5 days.

Orange Blossom Honey Syrup

Honey adds a complexity to cocktails that the standard simple syrup lacks. By adding warm water (here in a 2:1 ratio), the honey thins enough to blend seamlessly into a drink without diluting its flavor. Use honey syrup in the cocktails here or, if you substitute it in a recipe that calls for simple syrup, start by adding half the amount of syrup called for and adjusting to taste.

1 cup orange blossom honey

½ cup warm water

In a medium jar, combine the honey and warm water. Cover and shake until the honey dissolves. Store in the refrigerator for up to 1 month.

Bee's Knees

It seems silly to write a book on honey and not include this suitably-named and undeniably tasty cocktail. The original Bee's Knees recipe called for equal parts of lemon juice, honey and gin, but ready access to high-quality gin warrants a heavier pour.

Ice

2¼ ounces gin

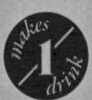

¾ ounce fresh lemon juice

¾ ounce orange blossom honey syrup (above)

Fill a cocktail shaker with ice. Add the gin, lemon juice and honey syrup; shake well. Strain into a chilled coupe and serve.

Brandy Slush

Every year, a few days before Christmas, my mom pulls out a massive plastic bucket and pours in a potent mixture of instant tea mix, frozen lemonade and orange juice concentrates and more brandy than one should serve at even the most raucous of parties. The result, frozen into slush and diluted with a splash of citrus soda, is a debaucherous treat that provides the ideal fix to get through social and family functions. This rendition is a hair more sophisticated than the tipple served back home, but it's just as rowdy.

2½ cups fresh orange juice

¾ cup orange blossom honey syrup (opposite)

½ cup fresh lemon juice

¼ cup high-quality maraschino cherries, finely chopped

2 tablespoons maraschino cherry juice

3 dashes Angostura bitters

¾ cup brandy

Seltzer water

serves
6

In a large bowl, whisk together the orange juice, honey syrup, lemon juice, cherries, cherry juice, Angostura bitters and brandy. Pour the mixture into a 9-by-13-inch metal pan.

Freeze, uncovered, for 1 hour. Use the tines of a fork to stir the mixture, scraping up and dispersing any icy bits. Return the pan to the freezer, scraping every hour or so, until the mixture is frozen and similar in texture to shaved ice, about 4 hours. Cover the dish in plastic wrap and keep frozen until ready to serve.

To serve, spoon some of the brandy slush into a lowball glass and top with seltzer. Serve immediately.

Mike's Honey-Vanilla Old-Fashioned

Mike, my stepdad, has been making old-fashioneds for as long as I can remember. Throughout the years, he's tweaked the whiskey proportions to get just the right amount of burn-to-sweet ratio. When developing the recipes for this book, I took a trip back home, slipped him a batch of honey syrup and a vanilla bean and let him go at it. He got it right on the first try, but we "retested" the cocktail all weekend long, just to be sure.

1½ ounces bourbon whiskey

½ ounce rye whiskey

¼ ounce orange blossom honey syrup (p. 40)

¼ vanilla bean, split and scraped

4 dashes Angostura bitters

Ice

1 orange twist, for garnish

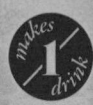

Combine the bourbon, rye, honey syrup, vanilla bean seeds and bitters in a mixing glass. Fill with ice and stir until chilled. Strain into an ice-filled rocks glass. Garnish with an orange twist and serve immediately.

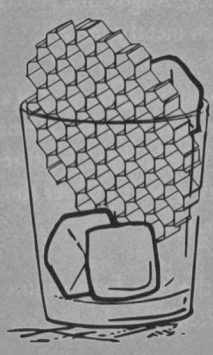

Switchel

A bracing blend of water, molasses, ginger and cider vinegar, switchel (also called haymaker's punch, switzel or swizzle) was the preferred late-summer quaff of 17th-century Colonists and 19th-century hay farmers. A precursor to sports drinks, the sweet-tart beverage both quenched thirst and replenished electrolytes. This rendition swaps in honey syrup for the molasses and adds lemon to lighten the flavors. The result is no less refreshing, whether you've spent the day tilling hay or doing something less taxing. Serve it as is or add a finger of rum for an even more fortifying tipple.

2 tablespoons orange blossom honey syrup (p. 40)

2 tablespoons apple cider vinegar

½ teaspoon finely grated ginger

2 tablespoons fresh lemon juice

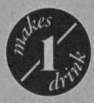

In a Mason jar, combine the honey syrup, vinegar, ginger and lemon juice. Add 1 cup of water, cover and shake to combine. Refrigerate until chilled; serve over ice.

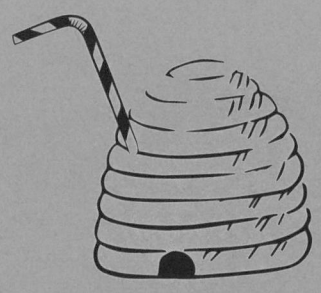

Switchel

A bracing blend of water, molasses, ginger and cider vinegar, switchel (also called haymaker's punch, swizzel or swizzle) was the preferred late-summer spirit of 19th-century Colonials and 19th-century boy farmers. A precursor to sports drinks, this sweet tart beverage quenched thirst and replenished electrolytes this rendition swaps in honey syrup for the molasses and adds lemon to lighten the flavor. Though the lemon isn't taxing, whether you've spent the day tilling hay or doing sun salutations, you'll savor a gradual ease of tension more than ever. You'll drink...

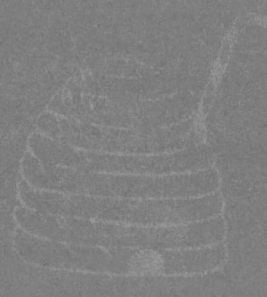

Thank You!

Special thanks to my beautiful mother for offering a week in her kitchen (with dishwashers!) and a lifetime of support. To Brett, for tackling months of honey-laced meals and countless sticky pots and pans with a hearty appetite and more enthusiasm than I deserve. To the Short Stack team for the incredible opportunity. And, last but not least, to the bees, without whom none of this would be possible.

—*Rebekah Peppler*

Share your Short Stack cooking experiences with us
(or just keep in touch) via:

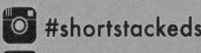 #shortstackeds
@shortstackeds

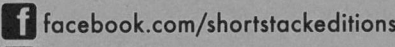 facebook.com/shortstackeditions
hello@shortstackeditions.com

Colophon

This edition of Short Stack was printed by The Print House in New York City on Neenah Astrobrights Galaxy Gold (interior) and Neenah Oxford White (cover) paper. The main text of the book is set in Futura and Jensen Pro, and the headlines are set in Lobster.

Sewn by:

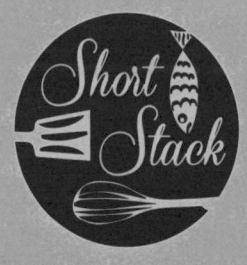

Available now at ShortStackEditions.com: